Dandelion
Medicine

A Medicinal Herb Guide

Dandelion Medicine

Remedies and Recipes to

- **Detoxify**
- **Nourish**
- **Stimulate**

Brigitte Mars,
Herbalist AHG

STOREY
BOOKS

Schoolhouse Road
Pownal, Vermont 05261

*The mission of Storey Communications is to serve our customers
by publishing practical information that encourages
personal independence in harmony with the environment.*

This book is intended to educate and expand one's concepts of how to deal
with a crisis. It is not intended to take the place of courses in first aid or to
replace medical care when needed.

Edited by Deborah Balmuth and Nancy Ringer
Cover design by Meredith Maker
Cover art production and text design by Betty Kodela
Text production by Mary Minella and Jennifer Jepson Smith
Illustrations by Sarah Brill, except as follows: Bobbi Angell, dedication page; Nancy
    Anisfield, page 94; Beverly Duncan, pages 46 (top), 50, 53, 54, 55, 58, 59, 60, 61,
    64; Brigita Fuhrmann, page 85; Regina Hughes, page 5; Nancy Hull, page 14;
    Charles Joslin, pages 46 (bottom), 48, 52 (top), 88; Alison Kolesar, pages 37, 49,
    74, 91, 93, 96, 101, 102; Randy Mosher, pages 43, 45, 67, 68
Indexed by Susan Olason, Indexes & Knowledge Maps

Printed in the United States by R.R. Donnelley
10 9 8 7 6 5 4 3 2

Library of Congress Cataloging-in-Publication Data

Mars, Brigitte.
        Dandelion medicine / Brigitte Mars.
                p.   cm. — (A medicinal herb guide)
        ISBN 1-58017-207-5 (pb : alk. paper)
        1. Dandelions—Therapeutic use.   I. Title.   II. Series.
    RM666.D26M37   1999
    615'.32399—dc21
                                                        99-33559
                                                        CIP

DEDICATION

To my beloved daughter,
Sunflower Sparkle Mars

CONTENTS

Dandelion!
Don't you be cryin'
We're doing our best to tell the world about you!
Sunshine bright
You ray of light
Concentrating solar energy
You are free
Growing all around me
Blessed be
Yeah God!
Ray of gold
I am told
Helps heal people and the planet
I do believe
It is time to perceive
The truth about weeds
That fulfill so many of our needs
Breathe deep the breath of life!
Hurrah, Dandy Lion!

— Brigitte Mars, 1998

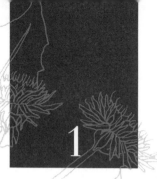

1

THE VIRTUES
OF THE DANDELION

Dandelions may well be the world's most famous weed. Each spring they burst into a carpet of sunny yellow blossoms. The flowers open wide to greet the morning and then close toward evening. To listen to the media, with all their ads for weed killers, however, you'd think that dandelions were a serious threat to humanity — when it's the herbicides that really do the harm! Every year, Americans spend millions of dollars on herbicides so that we may enjoy uniform lawns of nonnative grasses, and then use 30 percent of the nation's water supply to keep those lawns green. Meanwhile, those same herbicides poison our air, water, and ultimately our bodies.

Though dandelion today is considered by most people to be a useless weed, in truth it is one of the most beneficial and healthful of herbs. Every part of the dandelion has a use, ranging from food, to medicine, to dye. These beneficial properties did not always go unnoticed in North America: Up until the 1800s, people would actually pull the grass out of their yards to make room for dandelions and other useful "weeds" such as chickweed, malva, and chamomile.

As Ralph Waldo Emerson wrote, "What is a weed? A plant whose virtues have not yet been discovered." The time has come again to learn the virtues of the dandelion.

WHAT IS A DANDELION?

It has been said that the average American recognizes more than a thousand logos for commercial products, yet recognizes fewer than five plants that grow in his or her area. For most people, the dandelion is likely to be one of these familiar plants.

Botanical Origins

The botanical name for dandelion is *Taraxacum officinale*. The genus name, *Taraxacum*, is from the Arabic and means "bitter herb." It may have evolved from the Greek *taraxos*, a term used by Arab physicians of the early Middle Ages to mean "disorder," and *akos*, meaning "remedy." Or it could be derived from the Greek *taraxia*, meaning "eye disorder," and *akeomai*, "to cure," as dandelion was traditionally used as a remedy for the eyes.

The species name, *officinale*, tells us that the plant is or was an "official medicine," or "the plant of the apothecaries in Rome."

What's in a Name?

The word *dandelion* is a Saxon corruption of the Norman term *dent de lion*, meaning "tooth of the lion," perhaps a reference to the serrated leaves. Each of the florets has five toothed edges, another correlation to lion's teeth. Some say the comparison to lions has to do with the flower's bright yellow color; others say simply that the plant is as strong as the tooth of a lion. The name may also symbolize the traditional astrological connection between the sun and lions — Leo (the Lion) is governed by the Sun.

Dandy Nicknames

Dandelion has also been known by a variety of nicknames, including amarga, bitterwort, blowball, cankerwort, chicoria, clockflower, consuelda, devil's milkpail, doonhead clock, fairy clock, fortune-teller, heart-fever grass, Irish daisy, milk gowan, milk witch, monk's head, peasant's cloak, puffball, priest's crown, sun in the grass, swine's snout, tell-time, tramp with the golden head, piss-en-lit (meaning "pee in the bed"), piddly bed, wet-a-bed, yellow gowan, and wild endive.

Each of the names has historical or cultural significance. For example, *gowan* is a Scottish word for "daisylike flower." Names such as blowball and tell-time are reminders of a traditional game: Children blow the seed heads and watch them disperse and fly away; the number left is supposed to signify the hour. When the mature flower head closes, it resembles a pig's snout; hence the nickname swine's snout. The plant is sometimes known as monk's head — when all the seeds have gone, the top looks like a priest's tonsure, or shaved crown.

A DANDELION BY ANY OTHER NAME

Around the world dandelion is well known and named:
- Chinese — *chian-nou-ts'ao, huang-hua ti-ting*
- French — *piss-en-lit*
- German — *löwenzahn, kuhblume*
- Greek — *radiki* (meaning "radiating from the center")
- Hindi — *dudhal*
- Italian — *dente di leone*
- Japanese — *hokoei*
- Korean — *p'ogongyong*
- Mandarin — *pu gong ying*
- Persian — *trakhasnkun* ("bitter herb")
- Russian — *oduvanchik, pushki*
- Sanskrit — *dughdapheni*
- Spanish — *diente de león*
- Turkish — *kara hindiba otu, yabani*
- Welsh — *dant y llew*

BOTANICAL FEATURES

Dandelion is believed to be native to Greece and the Mediterranean regions of Asia Minor and Europe. It is a perennial member of the Asteraceae family, which is one of the largest groups of flowering plants and includes daisies, sunflowers, and calendula as well as lettuce and endive.

Leaves

Dandelion is considered by botanists to be a dicot — that is, a plant that bears two leaves from its germinating seed. The hollow, unbranched stems grow 2 to 18 inches high atop a rosette of shiny, hairless, coarsely toothed green leaves that are broader toward the top than at the base. The teeth of the leaves are usually directed downward. The leaves grow in a basal rosette — quite an ingenious botanical design, as the natural grooving of the leaves helps to steer water to the roots of the plant.

Flowers

The plant first blooms, one yellow flower head per plant, in early spring. The blossom, measuring ½ to 2 inches in diameter, is actually a compilation of about 150 florets, each a complete tiny tube-shaped ray flower in its own right with anthers and stigmas. Each floret has five tiny teeth on its edge.

The flowering season in the northern hemisphere, where dandelions are most common, is from April to June. The blossoms close early in the evening and during cloudy weather, perhaps to protect the nectar and pollen as well as to conserve heat during cold spring nights. Dandelions are very sensitive to temperature; they bloom more when the weather is cool and the blooms clear and disappear as hot summer arrives. Dandelion has one of the longest flowering seasons of any plant, and when a warm spell occurs in an off season, it is not unusual to see the pretty yellow flowers.

Underneath the flower is a green calyx with downward-curved outer bracts. When the blossoming cycle is complete, the flower head folds up for several days, with the calyx drawn into a cylindrical shape around the ripening ovaries, before reopening to reveal its parachute-topped seeds. Dandelion is considered apomict: It produces seeds without pollination or fertilization. This bisexual tendency enables many various forms of the plant to evolve, each differ from the other in minute ways. The seeds, borne on a circular ball, are known as acheniums. They bear a feathery pappus (or tuft) and are carried on the wind — often as many as 5 miles from their origin.

The ovule contains special cells that produce embryos that are identical to the parent plant. The long taproot issues from a short rhizome. All of the underground portions are dark brown on the outside, white on the inside. The root can grow up to a foot long and is milky white inside with a brown epidermis. The taproot allows the plant access to water deep in the earth so that it can survive dry spells. The entire plant contains a milky white juice.

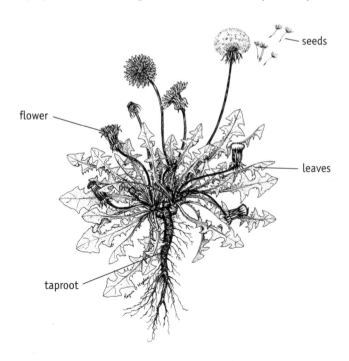

seeds

flower

leaves

taproot

Related Species

There are more than 150 useful species related to dandelion, including *Taraxacum magellanicum*, *T. erythrosperum* (red-seeded dandelion), *T. autumnalis* (fall dandelion or hawkbit), *T. ceratophorum* (horned dandelion), *T. eriophorum* and *T. scopulorum* (both Rocky Mountain dandelion), *T. ceratophyllum* (tundra dandelion), *T. lyratum* (dwarf alpine dandelion), and *Krigia virginica* (dwarf dandelion). To identify a dandelion cousin, remember that dandelions grow with an unbranching stem from a rosette of leaves. Any plant that has any branching characteristics is not a dandelion relation.

LORE AND LEGEND: HOW THE DANDELION CAME TO BE

Because dandelion can be found in many parts of the world, there are many different legends and folkloric stories explaining how the dandelion came to be. Dandelions also predominate in the traditional mythology of many cultures. For example, ancient Greek mythology tells the tale of Hecate, goddess of the earth and underworld, honoring Theseus with a salad of dandelion greens after he slew the infamous Minotaur.

Fairies and Wood Sprites

Following in the footsteps of many other creation stories, one popular legend ascribes dandelion's birth to the work of fairies. Many thousands of years ago, when the world was populated with fairies and elves, the first humans arrived. They soon caused these tiny creatures many problems, as the humans were usually unable to see the wee folk and would step on them. So the fairies took to dressing in bright yellow garments and eventually were changed into dandelions, which have the ability to spring back up if trodden upon. Thus, it is believed that dandelions recover so quickly from being stepped on because each contains the spirit of a fairy.

Another folkloric story tells of a miserly old man who discovered a pot of gold at the end of a rainbow. He decided to hide it in the ground rather than share his good fortune. In order to think about where he would bury it, he took the gold home with him in a sack and then went to bed. While he was sleeping, a hungry mouse, in search of food, gnawed a hole in the sack.

Early the next morning, the man grabbed the sack and went to bury it. As he reached a dark part of the forest, he noticed how light the sack had become. When he looked inside, there were but a few coins left. "My gold has fallen out!" he cried. "I shall retrace my steps and pick it all back up!" Believing the nuggets would be easy to spot on the ground, he walked back and bent down to collect the shiny gold pieces. However, they had become rooted to the ground. When he looked closer, he noticed that each coin was now a golden flower. Wood sprites had transformed the coins into golden flowers for all to enjoy.

Native American Stories

A Native American legend holds that once a beautiful, golden-haired maiden was admired by the South Wind. The South Wind was too lazy to court her, so he lay in the shade and watched her as she smelled the flowers. He waited so long that one day, when awakening from a nap, he noticed that she was now a gray-haired woman. The South Wind blamed his brother the North Wind, believing it was he who had blown a frost upon her to whiten her golden hair. To this day, the South Wind continues to sigh for the love he may have once enjoyed.

Another Native American legend involves a golden-haired girl who fell in love with the Sun. She rejected all suitors and simply watched the Sun make his journey across the sky, although he ignored her. She grieved until she got old, frail, and gray and was blown away by the wind. The Sun, finally noticing, felt sorry that he had not paid attention to her and could not bring her back. The Great Spirit took pity and sent small golden flowers to bloom on the prairies, and to this day the wind carries off the gray-haired seeds.

MAGIC AND MYSTERY

In the sixteenth century, Pier Andrea Mattioli, an Italian physician and author of *Commentarii in Sex Libros Pedacii Dioscorides,* wrote, "Magicians say that if a person rubs himself all over with dandelion, he will be everywhere welcome and obtain what he wishes." Rubbing your skin with dandelion juice was believed to ensure that you would receive hospitality in any home.

According to astrology, dandelion corresponds to the air element. It is governed by Jupiter and considered a masculine plant. Herbs ruled by Jupiter are cheerful, benevolent, soothing, and jovial. Dandelion is also under the dominion of the Sun, which governs plants of a bright golden color. In Ayurvedic medicine, however, dandelion is ruled by Saturn, which governs cool, bitter, and detoxifying herbs.

THE DOCTRINE OF SIGNATURES

The Doctrine of Signatures is a folkloric belief that plants give us hints as to what they are good for by the way they look. It has evolved from bits of astrology, alchemy, fact, and fantasy. The doctrine is founded on the belief that by observing a plant — the color of its flower, the shape of its leaf or root — you can determine its place in nature's plan. For example, the form of kidney beans tells us that they're good for the kidneys; blood-red beets fortify the blood; a head of cauliflower benefits the brain.

What Dandelion Tells Us

Dandelion is a survivor. It reaches deep into the earth, making it impervious to burrowing animals and fire. The bright yellow color of the flower corresponds to the liver and thus explains its use in treating gallstones and jaundice. Because dandelion has a juicy stem and root, it was considered beneficial for increasing urine production. The roots and leaves are associated with the physical body, the yellow flowers with mental health, and the puffball seed head with emotional well-being. As the seeds fly off and return to the earth, they represent the muscular structure being calmed.

The liver is an organ that has suffered numerous assaults from chemicals in our environment. So, too, the dandelion, yet it continues to adapt and also helps the human organism to adapt. Dandelion is indeed hardy. It grows through cracks in the sidewalks; thrives despite a multitude of herbicides; and can even withstand 20,000 volts of electricity. Where lawns are mowed, the dandelion keeps a very short stem, but in tall grass their stems stretch to greater height in order to catch the rays of the sun. If the leaves or flowers are cut, more grow back within a few days. It seems fitting that a plant that has adjusted so well to the environment can help humans adapt to a polluted planet — while we do our best to correct the situation. The simple abundance of the dandelion may perhaps be a sign that we should be using lots of this gift of nature!

Look Like Rain?

Dandelion flowers close up when it is about to rain, so next time you're wondering whether you need to bring along an umbrella, just check to see what your dandelion friends are doing.

Other Folklore Beliefs

There are so many wonderful facts and much mythology about this plant! Following are just a few bits of dandelion lore that have been passed down to me.

- Drinking a tea of dandelion leaves is said to promote psychic ability, especially if you drink the tea while visualizing an increase in that talent.
- Maidens would blow on the seed head; the number of seeds remaining would determine how many children they would have once they married.
- When a maiden blew on a dandelion seed head, if at least one seed remained, it was a sign that her sweetheart was thinking of her.
- When the downy seeds blow off the dandelion and there is no wind, it will rain.
- Lovers should blow dandelion seeds in the direction of their beloved to send messages of affection.
- Blow on a dandelion seed head and however many seeds are left are how many more years you will live.
- Make a wish and then blow on the seed head. If every single seed flies away, your wish will come true.
- Growing dandelions at the northwest corner of your property is said to bring favorable winds.
- In the Victorian language of flowers, dandelion signifies love. It is also a symbol of wishes, welcome, faithfulness, and divination. In some cultures it is considered good luck to dream of dandelions; in others, though, a dandelion dream portends ill fortune, indicating that the dreamer's lover was untrue.

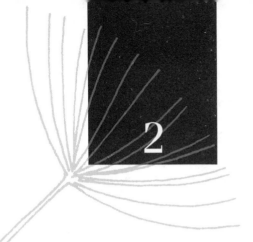

COLLECTING, GROWING, AND HARVESTING

Dandelions grow worldwide except in deserts and in the tropics. This herb seems to follow the steps of civilization and cultivation. It is especially prolific throughout the northern temperate zones and can flourish from sea level up to altitudes of 10,500 feet. There are even reports of a variety growing in the Himalayas at 18,000 feet!

BENEFITS FOR THE SOIL AND THE ENVIRONMENT

Dandelion grows where the soil is healthy — it is considered an indicator of the presence of potassium, magnesium, calcium, and sodium. Dandelions prefer loose, rich, well-drained, nitrogen-rich soil with neutral acidity, but they can tolerate a wide range of conditions. Because of dandelion's deep taproot, it doesn't compete with short-rooted grasses. The long roots help to aerate the soil, providing drainage channels for water, and help to heal barren or overworked soil by soaking up nutrients that have been washed downward and bringing them up toward the surface where other, shorter-rooted plants can use them — sort of like an

> *Where the Dandelion grows, the garden will flourish.*
>
> — OLD FARMERS' SAYING

herbal earthworm: facilitating, not competing. Dandelions also help to convert nitrogen to nitrates in the soil. They are a natural humus magnet, as earthworms enjoy the soil near them (hence the Chinese nickname, "earth nail").

Dandelion growing in fruit orchards gives off ethylene gas at sunset, which helps fruit to ripen early and evenly. Not only do the fruits grow larger, but so, too, do the dandelions. They seem to have a cooperative, symbiotic relationship.

When dandelions die, the channels formed by their roots open up the earth for other plants to grow. If uprooted dandelions are added to compost, they work as an activator, speeding up the decomposition of composted material; they also help provide copper as a nutrient.

A Friend to Creatures

Dandelion blooms in the spring, at a time when other sources of pollen are scarce. The stigma of the flower grows through the tube formed from the anthers. The stigma pushes the pollen forward, which coats visiting insects who then carry it to other flowers and thus ensure cross-pollinization. It has been reported that at least

---

SURVIVING ON DANDELION

Should you find yourself in a survival situation with nothing to eat except old dandelion greens, boil the leaves in two changes of water to remove the bitter flavor. The plant has even been used as survival food in polar regions.

Boy Scouts learn that even the seedlike fruits (found on the stem, at the base of the parachute), though somewhat bitter, can be eaten raw in an emergency — remove the plumelike hairs by rubbing the seeds in your palms to separate them from the stalks.

85 different insects are nourished by dandelions, including butter-flies, wasps, flies, and beetles. Bees love it — dandelion is an important plant for honey production.

Canada geese, grouse, pheasants, and many other birds eat the seeds. Purple finches are particularly attracted to dandelions. Leaves are consumed by black- and grizzly bears, chipmunks, elk, and porcupines. Goats, pigs, and rabbits will eat the whole plant. Feed dandelions to domestic rabbits, guinea pigs, and gerbils. When cows consume dandelion, they produce even more milk, though they may not relish the bitter flavor. Dandelions are a favorite food for pigs and chickens. Horses will eat dandelion greens and roots when they are cut and mixed with bran. The leaves are even fed to silkworms when their usual food, mulberry leaves, is scarce.

GROWING HABITS

Dandelions are abundant in meadows, in waste places, along roadsides, and, of course, in lawns. The plant frequently grows where the soil has been disturbed. You'll often find dandelion as a companion to plantain, clover, and alfalfa.

The dandelion leaves lie flat, so this herb usually remains unharmed by the lawnmower. If you try to pull up the herb, so long as a small portion of the root remains in the soil, another plant will emerge. While many plant species are being lost to industrialization and the building of housing developments and shopping centers where once there were meadows, dandelions thrive in disturbed or compacted soils and near roads and highways, and will even sprout up through the cracks in your sidewalk. This herb has shown a remarkable ability to adapt to environmental stress.

A bit of lawn, thickly starred with the glowing yellow blossoms, isn't in itself a bad picture....Why not accept the beauty and find an added joy in fecundity which gives to us without trouble or cost and generally in spite of ourselves?

— COUNTRY LIFE IN AMERICA, 1909

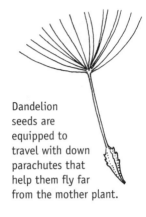

Dandelion seeds are equipped to travel with down parachutes that help them fly far from the mother plant.

I believe it wants to be here! It's time to change our attitude about dandelions in the lawn: Dandelions add to the beauty of a landscape with their cheerful, sunny flowers!

Dandelions are well suited to their own proliferation. Flowers form at the top of the root long before the final frost of winter, giving them the protection of several inches of soil and ensuring a long blooming season. The seeds are a type of flying apparatus with radiating threads that form a sort of parachute. When wind sweeps across, the seeds are, in the words of David Attenborough in *The Private Life of Plants*, like a "fragile elegant globe. Even the gentlest breath, from the wind or a child, can cause squadrons to take off and sail high and far through the sky." Seeds have been found as far away as 5 miles from their mother plant. Also, the seeds do not have to go through a long period before germinating; thus they need less time to grow than do many other plants.

CULTIVATING YOUR OWN

One hundred years ago, France produced seed catalogs that offered five varieties of dandelions. Given its versatility, it's not surprising that in many parts of the world, dandelion is cultivated and sold in the marketplace. We in North America are just catching on. Today, dandelion seeds are commercially available from many seed catalogs. You can also collect seed

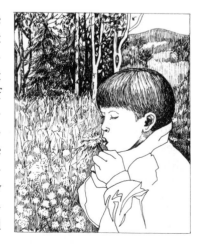

from the wild. To collect your own, cover the flowering plants with a piece of muslin to prevent the wind from carrying off the seeds. Collect the seeds in the evening, near sunset, when the dampness in the air causes the seed heads to close up. Store them in a cool, dry place in preparation for planting in late fall or early spring.

Sowing Seeds

It takes about 4 pounds of seed to grow one acre of the plant spaced at about 1 foot apart. This should yield enough seeds for four to five acres the second year, which will yield about 1,000 to 1,500 pounds of dandelion leaves.

Broadcast seeds directly in the ground. From a fall sowing, you will be able to enjoy the greens in spring. Seeds can also be sown directly in the ground in early spring (and they're quite hardy, so no need to wait for the last frost). Space the seeds about 12 inches apart and cover them with about ½ inch of soil.

> ### Organic Alert
>
> Dandelion is rarely attacked by disease or pests, making it a good candidate for organic gardening.

You can also start seed indoors. Sow the seeds in early spring on the surface of pots or divided plug trays. Cover with a fine layer of perlite. Avoid sowing in seed trays, as the long taproot will make it difficult to remove. Seeds germinate in three to six weeks. For container gardening, pots must be very deep to accommodate the long roots.

Root Division

Dandelion can also be propagated by root division. This method is best done in spring or fall where there is a cluster of dandelions. With a shovel, slice around the perimeter of a plant's root system and lift under the base of the plant, roots and all. By hand, divide the clumps of roots into smaller clumps and replant in another area. Water well.

GROWING TIPS

Dandelion is great for people who doubt their ability to grow anything, as it is a tenacious plant. Put in some dandelions — they'll
boost your green thumb confidence. Following are a few tips for
getting the most out of your crop.

- The wild plant is considered more medicinal than cultivated
  varieties. The cultivated plants have larger leaves and roots,
  however, and produce more leaves. Some people like to
  blanch the leaves by placing a flowerpot upside down over
  the growing plant. This reduces their nutritional content,
  though, as a dark green color indicates the presence of
  chlorophyll and carotenoids.
- Cultivated leaves tend to be thicker, more tender, and less
  bitter than those of the wild varieties, as well as lighter in
  color.
- If you are growing dandelion for a salad green, pick off the
  buds and prevent flowering to keep the greens from becoming bitter.
- To make a copper-rich garden fertilizer, pick three dandelion plants — roots, leaves, stems, and flowers — and place
  in a bucket with 1 quart (1 l) of boiling water. Let steep for
  ½ hour. Strain out and compost the spent plant material
  and use the liquid to water plants.
- In late fall, dig up dandelion roots, plant them in wooden
  crates of soil, and store in the basement or another cool,
  dark area. If watered regularly, you'll have blanched leaves
  throughout the winter, though blanching reduces the bitterness and decreases nutrient content.
- A trick for growing and harvesting your own dandelion
  roots is to plant the herbs on a narrow bed of loose soil to
  which some sawdust or wood chips have been added to
  make the soil more porous. Roots will then be easier to
  harvest.

HARVESTING DANDELIONS

It is likely that your neighbors will be delighted should you ask to collect dandelions from their lawns (providing their lawns haven't been sprayed). Be sure to gather from environmentally clean areas at least 50 feet away from busy roads and where no pesticides have been used. Roots will be easiest to harvest after a good rain or a few hours after the yard has been watered. If your neighbors don't live on a busy street and don't spray their lawns, ask permission to collect dandelions — then bring them some dandelion muffins to show your gratitude.

Should you live where dandelions simply don't grow, such as in a high-rise apartment building, check your local supermarket, farmers' market, or health-food store. Nowadays many retail grocery stores carry dandelions in their produce departments.

Leaves

Dandelion leaves are best collected in the spring before the plants flower. People who claim to dislike the taste of the greens have very likely collected the leaves after a plant has flowered, when the greens have turned bitter. If you wash the leaves before drying, be sure to dry them well to discourage mold. Cut the leaves at their base with a knife or snap them off with your fingers. After the plant has seeded, there will be a new growth of leaves later in the summer and these also can be collected. Avoid leaves that are yellow and wilted.

> The dandelion is the greatest natural agent of decoration in our part of America. In some fields it is so abundant that there is no more than enough grass visible to give to it a setting. It is so thoroughly at home that we feel it to be the most prominent and persistent native American, whatever its origin. Coming as it does in the early spring, it clothes an entire landscape with its gorgeous color and rejoices the heart of man . . . it is our tulip in the grass.
>
> — WALLACE NUTTING, CONNECTICUT BEAUTIFUL, PUBLISHED BY OLD AMERICA COMPANY, 1923

CASH CROP

Vineland, New Jersey, considers itself the Dandelion Capital of the World. The town grows close to half a million dollars' worth of this crop annually and holds a Dandelion Festival every year. Sales of fresh dandelion greens in the United States are estimated to be about $3 million. Arizona, California, Florida, and Texas are other states known for growing dandelions on a commercial scale.

Stems

The stems are best when the plant is in bloom. Stems are not commonly used as a food, but the sap they contain can be applied to warts to help make them disappear!

Flowers

When collecting flowers, it is helpful to have small children with you — they'll love to help. Spread the blossoms on a large cloth to allow some of the insects to crawl and fly away before you bring them inside. For appearance and efficacy, I recommend using the flowers the same day that they have been collected.

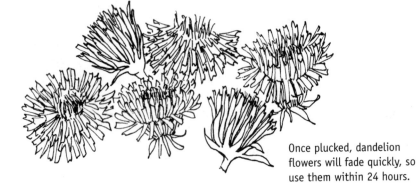

Once plucked, dandelion flowers will fade quickly, so use them within 24 hours.

Roots

There is a wonderful tool called a dandelion digger (available at gardening supply shops) that you can use for digging the deep dandelion taproots. To obtain large roots, gather plants that are at least 2 years old. The best roots will be found in unmowed patches of land and in soil that is rich and loose. Here the root is likely to be single and juicy. (In poorer soil, the root tends to be forked and tough.) The plant is most effective in its fresh state. Roots from older plants will be leathery to eat, but can still be used for medicine and in teas.

A dandelion digger is good for digging out any plant with a deep taproot, including the dandelion.

The ideal times to collect roots are in early spring before the plant flowers and then again in fall after the first frost.

Spring-harvested roots are sweeter than those taken in the fall, as they are higher in fructose and less bitter and fibrous. But they must be collected before the flower buds are big, or all of their energy will go into producing the blossom — this will deplete the root. From September to February is also an ideal time to collect the roots, when the plant is highest in inulin, which imparts a sweet taste. Spring roots are higher in taraxacin, which stimulates bile production, and fructose, a simple sugar, than fall roots.

Fall-harvested roots are more bitter and richer in inulin, which makes them more of a therapeutic medicine. This is partly because during the growing season, the fructose (also known as levulose) in the roots converts to inulin. The winter freeze then breaks down the inulin back to fructose, which sweetens the spring roots.

PRESERVING TECHNIQUES

There are many methods of preserving dandelions so that their nutritional and therapeutic benefits can be enjoyed through the cold winter months until they are available as fresh plants the next spring. Preserving dandelions thus gives you the opportunity to use this valuable plant year-round as food or medicine.

Drying Techniques

Drying herbs is an age-old technique that safely preserves the herb and creates an end product that is lightweight for carrying. Since drying evaporates the plant's water content, expect to have a lot less herb than what you started with.

Leaves. Rinse the leaves and blot dry. You can then place them in a food dehydrator or gather them in small bundles secured with a rubber band or string and hang them upside down in a dry, shady, well-ventilated location. Once crispy-dry, store the leaves in a glass jar in a cool, dark location. They should keep for one to two years.

Roots. Drying is the best method of preserving roots. To prepare the roots, scrub them well and slice the very largest roots lengthwise so that the insides will dry properly. Do not slice the roots before scrubbing, or the valuable milky juice will be washed away.

Once washed, place the roots on a screen and set in a cool, dry, shady, well-ventilated area. They should dry within 3 to 14 days, depending on the size of the roots and the humidity of the air. Alternatively, you can quick-dry them in an oven: Preheat the oven to 120°F and set the roots directly on the racks. Keep the door of the oven slightly ajar. Once dried (about 4 to 12 hours,

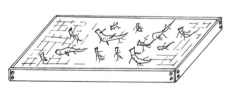

Set the screen in a dry, shady, well-ventilated area to encourage the roots to dry.

depending on the size of your roots), store the roots in a glass jar in a cool, dry place. They will keep for about a year.

Freezing

Collect greens (leaves) and wash them well. Steam them in a covered colander over a saucepan containing a few inches of boiling water for 1½ minutes. Then stop the cooking by plunging the greens into cold water. Put the greens into zip-seal bags, squeeze out the excess air, seal, and freeze. Frozen greens are suitable for use in recipes for cooked greens but should not be eaten raw.

GETTING RID OF DANDELIONS

The first crop of dandelions is a cheerful sign of spring. But perhaps your neighborhood association, unenlightened, is pressuring you to get rid of them. Share with a few neighbors some recipes and a copy of this book and start your own dandelion revolution! If this doesn't warm some hearts, remind people of the damage that herbicides cause to our planet. Spray programs are dangerous to animals and humans as well as to plants, and they poison our precious water supplies. Instead of chemicals, put some glitter in your yard — the golden flowers of the delightful dandelion.

Safe Alternatives to Herbicides

There are herbicides that have been developed for the sole purpose of killing dandelions. However, should you need to deter dandelions for some reason, instead of using toxic chemicals try mulching the area in which they grow with straw. Or apply black plastic to cover a weed-prone area — this will kill the plants underneath. The heat generated will destroy most weed seeds, too, as well as insects and disease organisms. Then avoid turning the soil; you don't want to bring a new crop of seeds to the surface.

You could plant something that will choke out the dandelions, such as rye or clover. Better yet — dig them up and use the roots for tea and food and make wine from the flowers! Dig up the plant when it is in flower, usually in April or May, before the seeds begin to form. At this point, the energy of the plant is aboveground and the food reserve in the root is less strong. If you leave a small piece of root in the ground, another dandelion will still come up. However, repeated diggings will eventually deplete the plant's food supply and cause it to lose its grip on life.

Tilling your dandelions under will only encourage more of them to grow. Instead, adjust the height of a lawnmower to 2½ to 3 inches (6.3 to 7.5 cm). The longer blades of grass will shade the dandelion leaves and stunt their growth. Or use a dandelion digger. This tool will make short work of removing dandelions you don't want.

Clipping the dandelion blossoms will discourage seeds from forming and thus decrease the plant's ability to spread. Use the harvested dandelion blossoms for food and medicine, of course.

A Final Plea

Isn't it time we learned to love and utilize the friendly dandelion? It offers itself freely, with something for everyone. Welcome this beautiful and useful plant. The people who tend to be the most aggressive about dandelions — angry, wanting to kill and rip things out of the earth — are probably the ones who could most benefit from this plant. Since you can't beat 'em, eat 'em — and enjoy the numerous health benefits.

Celebrate life and enjoy dandelions!

TRADITIONAL USES OF DANDELION MEDICINE

Dandelions have served humanity for thousands of years. The Greek naturalist Theophrastus (c. 732–287 B.C.) marveled at the dandelion's ability to flower over and over and recommended that the herb be taken as a tonic. In the Jewish tradition, dandelion leaves were one of the five bitter herbs of Passover mentioned in the Bible (Exodus). When Roman legions invaded Gaul and the Rhineland, they were delighted to find dandelions growing there. The Celts claimed dandelion as their own, relishing it to make food and wine. When Anglo-Saxon tribes settled in the British Isles after the withdrawal of the Romans, they used dandelion to prevent scurvy and as a diuretic and laxative.

EARLY WESTERN TRADITIONS

The Islamic physician Ibn sīnā (A.D. 980–1037) prescribed dandelion root to stimulate bile production for those with liver problems. It was the Arab physicians of this time who first described dandelion's diuretic properties.

Herbalists in thirteenth-century Myddfai, a village in Wales, wrote about the health benefits of dandelion. In a European herbal written in 1485 by Ortus Sannitatis, dandelion is mentioned as a medicinal plant. Nicholas Culpeper, an English herbalist of the seventeenth century, suggested dandelion for "every evil disposition of the body," which led to dandelion being considered "the official remedy for disorders." Culpeper also wrote of the dandelion: "You see here what virtues this common herb hath, and it is the reason the French and Dutch so often eat them in the spring; and now if you look a little farther, you may plainly see without a pair of spectacles, that foreign physicians are not so selfish as ours are, but communicative of the virtues of plants to people."

NORTH AMERICAN USES

Though the dandelion is not native to North America, it is believed that the plants may have arrived here with the Vikings in A.D. 100. It's just as likely that they arrived with early settlers, hitchhikers in vegetable seed packets, in the nineteenth century. Passengers on the *Mayflower*, however, intentionally carried dandelions across the sea with them.

LOVE CHARM

An Iroquois woman would select a dandelion with a particularly long taproot that had a fork and a small appendage resembling a part of the male anatomy. Then the name of her intended beloved was spoken several times and the root thrown behind her to ensure that her love soon would follow. Also as a love charm, dandelion roots that were found growing entwined would be boiled in water. When the water cooled, it was splashed on the face to make the user sexually irresistible.

Native Americans

The Native Americans welcomed this herb and gathered it for food and medicine. The Apaches collected it for days before their spring feasts. The Digger Indians of Colorado and the Papago of the Southwest ate dandelions both raw and cooked. The Iroquois boiled the leaves with fatty meats.

Many Native American tribes also used dandelion medicinally. An example: The Mohegans drank a tea of dandelion leaf as a liver tonic. Kiowa women boiled dandelion flowers with pennyroyal leaves to treat menstrual cramps. The Papago, too, used a tea of the flowers for menstrual cramps. The Navajo made a tea of the root for a new mother following birthing to hasten the delivery of the placenta. The Bella Coola of British Columbia and the Ojibwa both used dandelion root as a remedy for stomachache and heartburn. Delaware Indians used a dandelion root tea as a laxative and tonic. For the Mohegans and Potawatomi, the root was taken as a tonic tea. The Iroquois used dandelion to treat jaundice. The Fox Indians used a tea of the root to treat chest pains. The Tewa used a poultice of the leaves to help heal broken bones, bruises, swellings, sores, and fractures. Several tribes applied the juice from the stem to bee stings. The flowers also were used to make a yellow dye for deerskin.

> ## Heartburn Remedy
>
> Here's a common remedy from the Native American tradition for treating heartburn: Boil a handful of flowers until the water turns yellow, leave it to steep overnight, and give first thing in the morning; continue treatment for one month.

Many tribes chewed various plants as a gum to moisten their mouths. Dandelion stems, because of their latex content, were used in this way. The young plant was regarded by many tribes as having mild narcotic properties, too.

Early American Colonists

By the time the Puritans set sail for America, dandelion was considered an essential food and a health-giving plant. As European colonists settled along the Atlantic coast, they brought dandelion seeds with them to grow in their gardens. By 1630 dandelions were everywhere around the Plymouth Colony. Pioneer women actually raised dandelions to remind them of home, and fenced the precious plants to keep out gophers. As forests were cut down, dandelion seeds escaped to grow where room was now abundant.

Pioneer women considered dandelion an ally and never had a thought that they were a nuisance. During the Civil War, both North and South used it as food and medicine, especially when regular food supplies were cut off by blockades. They also substituted the roasted roots for coffee, and continued to do so even after the war. In the 1800s, settlers in the Midwest introduced the dandelion to provide food for bees, and dandelion's spread across the continent continued.

Twentieth-Century Traditions

Dandelion was an official herb in the early *Pharmacopoeia* of the United States. The root was considered the significant part of the plant from 1831 to 1926 and was included in the *National Formulary* until 1965.

*Star-disked Dandelion,
just as we see them,
Lying in the grass, like
sparks that have leapt
From kindling suns
of fire.*

— OLIVER WENDELL HOLMES,
"DANDELION,"
PROFESSOR AT THE
BREAKFAST TABLE

Dandelion is still included in the pharmacopoeias of Hungary, Poland, Russia, and Switzerland. Russians referred to dandelions as "the elixir of life," and it was a favorite remedy of the imperial court from the time of Peter the Great until the early 1900s. In rural Russia, dandelion root is still used to treat tuberculosis and prevent miscarriage.

During World Wars I and II, health departments in both the United States and

DANDELION EUPHEMISMS

There is a French expression that translates to "eating dandelion by the roots," which means the same as the American expression "pushing up daisies": it implies that someone is dead.

Europe publicized this herb as a healthful food. Before World War I, dandelions were cultivated in Germany and the roots that were exported were as large as parsnips. By World War II, England had stopped growing many herbs, feeling it was cheaper to import them, yet when their supplies were cut off, the British Ministry of Health organized teams of women to collect dandelions. Honored for its war service, dandelion was given a place in the British *Pharmacopoeia*.

During World War II, when many people suffered nutritional deficiencies, Italian housewives in small villages would brew up a pot of dandelion soup and leave it on a windowsill as nourishment for those passersby who were poor. Dandelion flowers were also chopped and added to spreads to give the appearance of butter.

Throughout the twentieth century and in popular culture today, there have been many other uses devised for dandelion from a wide range of cultures for a vast range of purposes:

- Lydia Pinkham, the great Quaker nurse, herbalist, and businesswoman of the mid-nineteenth and early twentieth centuries, included dandelion root in the original recipe for her famous women's tonic.
- The Eclectic physicians of the early 1900s, who combined herbal and modern medicine, regarded dandelion as beneficial for autointoxication (clearing toxins out of the body).
- In Japan, dandelions are cultivated as an ornamental plant. The Japanese have produced two hundred colorful varieties in white, orange, copper, and black.

- A popular Dutch legend says that if you eat dandelion salad on Mondays and Thursdays, you will be healthy always.
- Dandelions have long been a favorite spring vegetable of the Mennonites and the Amish peoples.
- The Pennsylvania Dutch have a custom of eating a bowl of dandelion greens on Green Thursday, in the belief that eating them on that day will ensure good health the rest of the year.

DANDELION IN CHINESE MEDICINE

Dandelion grows abundantly in China, especially in the Yangtze River valley, and records from the Tang dynasty date its use back to at least the seventh century. In China, a related species, *Taraxacum mongolicum*, which they call *pu-gong-ying*, is used to "clear heat" or treat infections or "fire poisons" as well as to clear dampness. The Chinese also call their dandelion *huang-hua ti-ting*, meaning "yellow-flowered herb," or *chian-nou-ts'ao*, meaning "plowing and hoeing weed."

Organizing on Its Behalf

Until the twentieth century, there existed a National Dandelion Society. Maybe it's time for a comeback. In the past decade, England has expressed concern over the possibility of the dandelion becoming extinct because of herbicide use, which has prompted the Save the Dandelion Society. See Sources for information on joining the North American version, Defenders of the Dandelion.

The Liver System

In traditional Chinese medicine, dandelion is often used to treat the Liver, which governs circulation of Blood and is important in maintaining a smooth flow of *chi*, or life energy, through the body. Dandelion tea made from the entire plant is used for any "hot" disorder that manifests in excess "heat" in the Liver.

According to Chinese medicine, the liver system is associated with anger and depression. As you begin to use dandelion, stored emotions that you thought you had forgotten may arise and become stirred up before leaving your body. On the other hand, dandelion root can be prescribed to clear stored, negative emotions.

The Herb for All Seasons

Dandelion is officially recognized in the *Pharmacopoeia* of the People's Republic of China, and practitioners of Chinese medicine have used dandelion to treat an incredible assortment of ailments and illnesses, including:
- Abscesses, boils, carbuncles, and sores
- Appendicitis
- Breast problems such as cancer, lack of milk production, mastitis, and tumors
- Chronic pelvic inflammatory disease
- Colds, fevers, and pneumonia
- Coughs and bronchitis
- Dental problems
- Eye inflammation
- Food poisoning
- Hemorrhoids
- Hepatitis
- Inflammation of the gums, mouth, and throat
- Insect bites
- Itchy skin
- Jaundice
- Mumps
- Pancreatitis
- Snakebites
- Tonsillitis
- Ulcers

AYURVEDIC MEDICINE

Ayurveda, translated as "life science," is the traditional system of healing in India and is now rapidly gaining popularity worldwide. It's based on mind-body-spirit connections that address specific body and energy types. In Ayurveda, dandelion is considered an herb that helps to purge *ama* (accumulated waste and toxins) from the body. It nurtures the air element *(vata)* and decreases fire *(pitta)* and water *(kapha)*, and thus should be used with caution by those with extreme vata constitutions. As in Chinese medicine, dandelion is thought of as bitter, sweet, and cooling.

Specific Uses

In Ayurvedic practice, dandelion is used for stagnation of energy in the liver and gallbladder and helps to cleanse bile ailments as well as breast problems such as tumors, insufficient milk production, cysts, and swollen lymph glands. Dandelion leaf is used most often for acute conditions and the root for chronic conditions, such as boils, carbuncles, gout, and cancer.

Ayurvedic medicine holds that dandelion is safe and beneficial for appetite loss and poor digestion, as it improves assimilation. It is also used for gynecological problems such as pelvic inflammatory disease and endometriosis. It is considered astringent, strengthening to the entire body, a cooling energy tonic, and beneficial in treating infection.

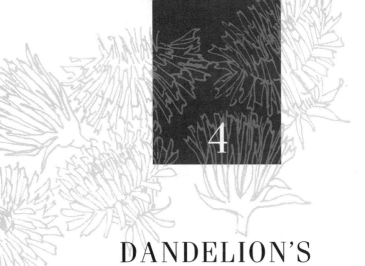

DANDELION'S
MEDICINAL PROPERTIES

As a medicinal plant, *Taraxacum* is a self-contained pharmacy. It is one of the most widely used herbal medicines in the world. The systems primarily affected by dandelion are the liver, kidneys, gallbladder, pancreas, intestines, and blood. It is held in particularly high regard as one of the safest and most important herbs for the liver.

Dandelion root is most medicinal in the unroasted form and may be taken in a tea, in an extract, or in capsule form. Leaves are also commonly used as medicine and may be used fresh or dried in the form of tea, tincture, and capsules. Fresh stems provide the sap, which also has medicinal properties. The flowers are best used fresh and are used mainly as a food source.

A CURE-ALL FOR WHAT AILS YOU

Dandelion has been used to cure just about everything at some time and in some place. The leaves, with their mineral-rich properties, can be used for nourishing our bones (warding off osteoporosis) and our teeth. Drinking dandelion leaf tea over time helps to increase joint mobility and reduce stiffness; decrease

> ## Dandelions for Better Sight?
>
> In the body, the beta-carotene from dandelion greens is converted to 11-cis retinol, the most important constituent of rhodopsin, a protein in the retina's rods (the cells that enable us to see in low-light conditions).

serum cholesterol and uric acid; and promote digestive regularity. Drinking a tea of the roots following birthing aids in the expulsion of the placenta. In Germany, dandelion juice from the stem and root are used to improve eye health — the plant is sometimes referred to as eye root. The Chinese use dandelion leaf internally to treat styes and conjunctivitis. Dandelions have long been used in cancer treatment; they are rich in chlorophyll and antioxidants like beta-carotene and flavonoids.

Giving Life to the Liver

Dandelion is a time-tested detoxifier and strengthener of the liver. In Germany, an over-the-counter drug called Hepatichol, which is made primarily from dandelion, is available for liver and gallbladder problems, including gallstones. Because the liver is the organ responsible for breaking down and clearing excess hormones from the body, one of the reasons that dandelion can improve menstrual problems is related to enhanced liver function.

Dandelion root is rich in phytosterols, so it is also excellent to use during menopause to alleviate hot flashes. It helps the liver break down excess luteinizing hormones and follicle-stimulating hormones. A woman going through menopause and using hormone replacement therapy can take dandelion to help nourish, protect, and support the liver while taking drugs.

Like other herbs that have an effect on the liver, dandelion helps to relieve anger, depression, jealousy, oversensitivity, and resentment. So think of this plant as both physically and emotionally beneficial: so much healing power with no harmful side effects!

CLINICAL TRIALS
AND SCIENTIFIC FINDINGS

Clinical studies to introduce a new drug often cost over 300 million dollars and are thus only affordable to large pharmaceutical companies, who hope to regain their expenditure when the new drug is released for sale. Understandably, then, there haven't been many studies on the medicinal value of an herb that grows so wild and free and is almost always readily available. However, dandelion has been used by millions of people for thousands of years! And over the past 100 years, the studies that have been conducted have served to confirm dandelion's beneficial properties.

Dandelion is known for its effects on the liver. This is due primarily to its ability to increase bile production by causing the gallbladder to contract, releasing stored bile and its high choline content, which acts as a tonic for the liver. As author and herbalist Christopher Hobbs reports, in a 1938 Italian study 12 subjects suffering liver dysfunction symptoms such as jaundice and low energy were injected with 5 milliliters of dandelion extract daily for 20 days. Cholesterol and urinary bilirubin were measured before and after administering the dandelion. Although the standards for testing are much more vigorous in modern times, 11 of the 12 subjects enjoyed a significant lowering of cholesterol levels and all 12 reported feeling better.

According to K. Faber, author of "The Dandelion," clinical trials in China from the mid-1900s proved dandelion to be effective against bronchitis, pneumonia, tonsillitis, and other respiratory disorders.

In a 1950 study conducted by L. Krroeber in England, dandelion was a successful remedy for hepatitis, jaundice, and liver enlargement, all common symptoms of liver dysfunction.

Dandelion has a long tradition of being a weight-loss herb for humans, which prompted researchers to study these claims on animals. In 1974, in a Romanian study by Elizabeth Racz-Kotilla, Gabriel Racz, and A. Solomon, rats and mice were given

50 milliliters of a dandelion infusion per every kilogram of body weight for one month. During this period they lost as much as 30 percent of their original weight. The loss was due to the diuretic activity of dandelion, the mild laxative effect, and the enhancing of liver function. It is also assumed that part of dandelion's weight loss–enhancing effect comes from its gland-stimulating qualities.

According to a 1979 study from Japan by K.K. Kotobuki Seiyaku, when the polysaccharide and aqueous extracts of dandelion have been administered to animals, they exhibit antitumor activity.

In *Chinese Materia Medica*, Dan Bensky, Andrew Gamble, and Ted Kaptchuk detail studies in China that indicate that dandelion has in vitro antibacterial effects against *Staphylococcus aureus, Streptococcus pneumoniae, Pseudomonas aeruginosa, Shigella* species, *Corynebacterium diphtheriae,* and *Neisseria meningitidis.*

Dandelion and its constituent inulin have shown positive hypoglycemic activity — helping to stabilize blood sugar levels — in animals. Inulin is composed of chains of fructose, which may possibly act to buffer the blood's levels of glucose and prevent sudden fluctuations.

Why Aren't There More Studies?

Why isn't more research conducted to prove the efficacy of this time-tested plant used by many world cultures? Well, as stated earlier, it's extremely expensive to introduce a new drug onto the market, and because dandelion proliferates just about everywhere, there's not much profit to be found in studying the plant for its possible uses as a drug. You can't patent a dandelion. Who would benefit if everyone could gather his or her own medicines? Certainly not the drug companies. Only the people and perhaps the planet as we stop spraying to eradicate this useful medicinal plant.

MEDICINAL PROPERTIES OF DANDELION

It would be difficult to think of a plant exhibiting more medicinal properties than does the dandelion. Here are some of its amazing effects.

PLANT PART	PROPERTY	ACTION/EVIDENCE
Root, leaf	Alterative	Help to purify the blood by increasing blood flow to the tissues, aiding assimilation and stimulating metabolism.
Root	Antibilious	Helps to remove excess bile from the system.
Root	Anti-inflammatory	Reduces inflammation, such as glandular swelling.
Leaf, sap, flower	Anodyne	Lessen nerve excitability, thus relieving pain.
Leaf	Antacid	Relieves stomach acid.
Root	Antibacterial	Inhibits the growth of germs.
Root, sap	Antifungal	Inhibit fungal growth.
Leaf	Antilithic	Helps to prevent and discharge urinary and biliary stones and gravel.
Leaf	Antioxidant	High in beta-carotene and vitamin C; helps the body resist free-radical damage.
Leaf, root	Antirheumatic	Root helps to disperse acidic deposits in the joints; leaves help gout and rheumatism as well as glandular swellings.
Leaf, root	Antitumor	Although there is not much data, dandelion has traditionally been used as a poultice to reduce tumors; in traditional Chinese medicine, dandelion poultices are used to treat breast cancer.
Leaf, root	Aperient	Work as a mild laxative.
Leaf, root	Astringent	Tighten and tone tissue. Help dry excessive secretions.
Leaf, root	Bitter	Stimulate the initial stages of digestion, including increasing saliva production and gastric juice activity as well as bile release.
Flower	Calmative	Mildly tranquilizing.
Flower	Cardiotonic	Benefits the heart.
Root	Cholagogue	Causes the gallbladder to contract and release stored bile from the liver. Can be used in cases of congestion of the liver and gallbladder.
Root	Choleretic	Stimulates bile production and increases cleansing of the bile duct.

(continued on next page)

MEDICINAL PROPERTIES OF DANDELION (continued)

PLANT PART	PROPERTY	ACTION/EVIDENCE
Leaf	Decongestant	Helps open respiratory passages and improve breathing.
Root	Deobstruent	Used to move obstructions, especially those originating in the liver.
Leaf, root	Depurative	Help to cleanse and purify the body.
Root, sap	Discutient	Help to dissolve abnormal growths.
Leaf, root	Digestive	Increase hydrochloric acid levels in the stomach. All the glands in the digestive system respond quickly to dandelion.
Leaf, root	Diuretic	Stimulate the flow of urine, so help reduce fluid retention. Helpful in cases of fluid retention due to heart problems.
Flower	Emollient	Used externally to soothe, soften, and protect the skin.
Leaf	Febrifuge	Helps lower fever.
Leaf, root	Galactagogue	Increase mother's milk.
Root, flower	Hepatic	Strengthen and tonify the liver.
Root	Hypnotic	Induces a deep, healing sleep state.
Leaf, root	Immune stimulant	Can be used for acute infections such as tonsillitis and pelvic inflammatory disease.
Root	Lipotropic	Prevents the accumulation of fat in the liver by stimulating bile production.
Root, leaf	Lithotriptic	Help to dissolve and discharge urinary and gallbladder stones.
Leaf	Laxative	Increases bowel function.
Leaf	Narcotic (mild)	Helps to relieve pain and induce sleep.
Leaf	Nutritive	Supplies lots of nutrients; builds and tones the body.
Root	Purgative	Increases bile secretions that activate intestinal peristalsis.
Root, leaf	Restorative	Help in the renewal and repair of organs and can help prevent further destruction. Also restorative to connective tissue.
Root	Sedative	Quiets the nerves.
Leaf, root	Stomachic	Strengthen and tonify the stomach. Improve digestion and relieve gas.
Leaf, root	Tonic	Promote general health and well-being.
Leaf, flower	Vulnerary	Encourage wound healing by promoting cellular growth and repair.

CONTRAINDICATIONS AND CAUTIONS

For most people, dandelion is considered safe even in large amounts; however, as with anything else, there is always the possibility that you could be allergic to it. There are no reports of toxic effects from its internal or external use. Even pregnant women use dandelion leaves, to prevent edema and hypertension. There have been very few cases reported of abdominal discomfort, loose stools, nausea, and heartburn associated with dandelion.

Kommission E, a German panel of experts on drugs and medical devices, allows dandelion leaf and root for their diuretic effects, as a cholagogue and appetite stimulant, and for dyspepsia, and they are an approved over-the-counter-drug. The German Kommission E feels dandelion to be contraindicated for obstruction of the bile duct, and suggests that it be used for gallstones only after consulting with a physician. In the United States, dandelion is considered *GRAS* (Generally Regarded as Safe); in the United Kingdom, dandelion is on the General Sales list; in Canada it is approved as an over-the-counter-drug; and in France it is classified as a Traditional Medicine.

> ### Caution
>
> Avoid using dandelions from lawns that have been sprayed with herbicides or chemical fertilizers in the past two or even three years.

The fresh latex in the stems can cause contact dermatitis is some sensitive individuals. Consult with a physician prior to using dandelion if you suffer from an obstructed bile duct or gallstones. Some individuals with gastric hyperacidity may find excessive use of dandelion leaf aggravating. To modify some of the cooling and contracting effects of dandelion when it is used over a long period, mix it with a small amount of ginger and licorice root. Truly, the chemicals used to poison this magnificent plant are far more dangerous than this herb ever could be!

Cautions for Children

Children delight in weaving crowns of the golden blossoms and blowing the fluffy seed heads. However, dandelion flowers wilt quickly once picked and do not make a good bouquet. If you place them in water, the flowers close up tightly. Children have become nauseous from sucking or eating too many dandelion flowers. Occasionally a child assimilates the diuretic properties through the skin from overhandling the fresh plant and thus may need to urinate more. Simply give the child a tea of peppermint, fennel seed, and chamomile, and he or she will begin to feel better.

BENEFITS FOR SPECIFIC AILMENTS AND CONDITIONS

Dandelion is often regarded as a blood purifier, which aids in the process of filtering and straining wastes from the bloodstream. It is useful in treating obstructions of the gallbladder, liver, pancreas, and spleen. The vulnerary, tonic, astringent, and antimicrobial properties of dandelion also make it helpful in the treatment of prostate problems. The leaves aid in the elimination of uric acid. Use the root primarily for problems related to the liver, spleen, stomach, and kidneys and the leaf for liver, kidney, and bladder concerns. Dandelion helps hypertension by decreasing excessive fluids in the body that the heart must pump.

During Pregnancy

When dandelion leaves are ingested during pregnancy, they strengthen the liver and can help prevent preeclampsia, which manifests as high blood pressure with edema. It helps the fetus to develop a strong liver of its own. Being high in iron, the leaves can help prevent anemia, a common concern for pregnant mothers.

High blood pressure and fluid retention during pregnancy can both be safely treated with dandelion leaf tea (and improvement in diet).

For Children

Taking dandelion root in the last few weeks of pregnancy will help prevent pathological jaundice in the baby. Should the baby have jaundice, the root — taken as a tea — ideally can be drunk by the nursing mother, or given to the infant directly as the next-best choice. About 1 teaspoon (5 ml) of the tea daily is appropriate for a baby, but the mother can drink as much as she is able. As dandelion leaf is a galactagogue, it increases the nursing mother's milk supply and bolsters its nutritional quality — another boon for the infant! The leaves and root of dandelion make an excellent food or tea rich in minerals for growing children. Because dandelion leaves and roots help to cleanse the liver, kidneys, and therefore the blood, they are excellent for teenagers concerned about acne.

FOR SIMPLE DELIGHT

For recreation, children's favorite pastime is to make chains of dandelions as necklaces, bracelets, and crowns. They also often strip the stems of flowers and leaves, split the stems at top and bottom, and then drop them in water to watch them curl and twist into pretty shapes.

AILMENTS EASED BY DANDELION REMEDIES

The following ailments can be helped by using dandelion in the form of a tea, tincture, capsule, or tablet. A general therapeutic dose is one cup of tea, one dropperful of tincture, or two 500-mg capsules or tablets three times daily. Please, in cases of serious illness, consult your health-care provider!

AILMENT	PLANT PART	AILMENT	PLANT PART
Abscess	root	Debility	fresh greens
Acne	root	Depression	root, flower
Age spots	root	Diabetes	root, leaf, stem
Alcoholism	root	Dizziness	root
Allergies	leaf, root	Dropsy	leaf
Amenorrhea	leaf	Dyspepsia	root, leaf
Anemia	leaf, root	Eczema	root, stem
Anorexia	leaf, root	Edema	leaf
Appetite loss	leaf	Endometriosis	root, leaf
Arthritis	root	Fatigue	leaf, root
Backache	flower, leaf	Flatulence	leaf, root
Bedwetting	leaf, taken earlier in the day	Gallbladder inflammation	leaf, stem
Boils	root	Gout	root helps to neutralize uric acid in the bloodstream
Breast tenderness, cysts, and breast cancer	root, leaf		
		Hangover	leaf, root
Bronchitis	leaf, root	Hayfever	root
Cancer prevention	leaf, root	Headache	root, flower
Candida	leaf, root	Heartburn	root
Cellulite	leaf, root	Hemorrhoids	root
Chickenpox	root	Hepatitis	root
Cirrhosis	root	Herpes	root
Cholesterol, high	root, leaf	Hypertension	root, leaf
Colitis	leaf, root	Hypochondria	leaf, root
Computer stress	leaf, root	Hypoglycemia	root
Congestive heart failure	leaf, root	Insomnia	leaf
Constipation	root	Jaundice	root

AILMENTS EASED BY DANDELION REMEDIES (continued)

AILMENT	PLANT PART	AILMENT	PLANT PART
Liver and gallbladder obstruction	root, stem	Prostatitis	leaf, root
		Psoriasis	root
Mastitis	leaf, root	Rashes	root, stem
Measles	root	Scrofula	leaf
Menstrual cramps	flower, root	Scurvy	leaf
Mononucleosis	leaf, root	Sinusitis	leaf
Morning sickness	root	Spleen enlargement	leaf, root
Mumps	root	Stomachache	leaf
Muscular rheumatism	leaf	Tonsillitis	leaf, root
Nervousness	leaf	Tuberculosis	root
Night blindness	flower	Tumor	root
Obesity	leaf, root	Ulcer	leaf, root
Osteoarthritis	root	Urinary tract infection	leaf
Ovarian cysts	root	Uterine fibroids	leaf, root
Poison oak and ivy	leaf, root	Varicose veins	root
Premenstrual syndrome	root	Venereal warts	root
Premenstrual water retention	leaf		

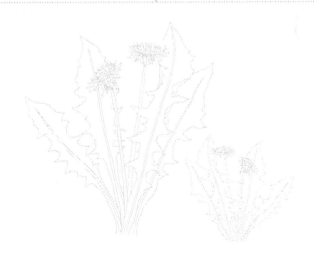

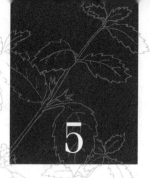

MAKING AND USING
DANDELION MEDICINES

There are many benefits to dandelion medicine. It's safe, effective, abundant, fresh, and free! It's pleasant to use and has a safety record that spans thousands of years of use. Medicinally, dandelions can be used fresh or prepared as a tea, tincture, encapsulated powder, juice, or homeopathic formula. Most dandelion remedies are easy to make at home, and in most regions, the fresh flowers are easy to collect — even, in fact, difficult to avoid tripping over. However, if you have neither the time nor the inclination, you can usually purchase harvested plants, dried leaves and roots, or remedies from health-food stores, herb shops, or mail-order sources (see Sources).

TEA PREPARATIONS

One of the greatest pleasures is a peaceful, reflective moment spent with a cup of tea. Taking the time to sit quietly over a cup of herbal tea, alone or with loved ones, is psychologically de-stressing, relaxing, and life-affirming; in addition, herbal tea is itself extremely healthful and can be healing as well. Think "I'm nourishing myself with the strength of this herb" as you savor any one of the following recipes. Beginning on page 46 are a number of healthful herbal formulas that utilize the benefits of dandelion. For medicinal purposes, drink three or four cups daily.

Making Infusions

To make a tea from the leaves of plants, there are two methods you can choose from. The glass-jar method takes longer but produces a stronger tea. The French-press method is quicker but not as strong. In both cases, use ½ ounce of dried leaves or 1 ounce of fresh leaves per cup of water. After straining, compost the spent leaves.

Glass-Jar Method: Place the tea ingredients in a glass canning jar. Cover with freshly boiled water. Put on the lid and allow to steep overnight, then strain out the solids.

French-Press Method: Simply place the herbs in a French press and cover with 1 quart of boiling water. Allow to steep for at least 20 minutes. (If you don't own a French press, first steep the herbs, then strain the tea through a non-aluminum strainer.)

The glass-jar method takes time but makes a potent tea.

THE DANDELION "CURE"

In Europe, many people commonly follow "the cure," which entails drinking three cups of dandelion root tea daily for six to eight weeks. They may do this twice a year, spring and autumn. Another spring cure is to take 1 or 2 tablespoons of dandelion leaf juice in some water morning and night for several weeks. In the fall a bit of juniper juice is also used when treating arthritic conditions. Consuming dandelion in the spring helps to counter the ill effects of a winter of eating only cooked, heavy foods. Drink dandelion leaf and root tea when on a cleansing diet or fasting.

Making Decoctions

A decoction is similar to an infusion, but is used to extract constituents from tougher, more fibrous parts of plants, such as roots,
tubers, barks, and woody stems. A decoction is necessary to
extract the healing properties from the roots of dandelion. Put 1
ounce of chopped dried roots or 2 ounces of chopped fresh roots
in a pan with 1 pint of water. Bring to a boil, cover, and simmer
for 20 minutes. Strain (you can compost the spent roots).

Combination Teas

When making a tea from both leaves, which require an infusion,
and roots, which require a decoction, first prepare the roots as a
decoction, as instructed above. After the 20 minutes of simmer-
ing, remove the pan from the heat, add the leaves, cover, and allow
the mixture to steep for at least 10 minutes. Now you have a
combination infusion-decoction. Strain out and compost the
spent herbs.

MAKING HERBAL TINCTURES

Tinctures are small and portable, making them easy to use when
you are at work, school, or traveling. For medicinal purposes, use
30 drops in a bit of hot water three times daily.

Both dandelion leaves and roots can be made into a tincture
using 1 part dandelion per every 5 parts of a 25 percent alcohol
solution, such as vodka or brandy. It makes sense to prepare
enough tincture to last at least a month, using an ounce as your
"part." In addition, any of the tea formulas that follow can easily
be made into a tincture. Prepare the herbs by chopping or grind-
ing (in a blender). Pour the formula into a jar large enough to
hold your herbs with some extra room. Cover with vodka or
brandy, adding an extra inch of the liquor so that the herbs are

saturated and completely covered. This will help to preserve the herbs and extract both the water-soluble and the alcohol-soluble proper-ties. Shake daily. Strain after a month, first with a strainer and then through a clean undyed cloth, squeezing tightly. Pressing the herbs with a potato ricer, while still in the cloth, can be helpful. Compost the spent herbs and bottle the tincture in dark glass containers. Label and date. Store away from heat and light. Tinctures will keep for 2 to 3 years.

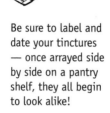

Be sure to label and date your tinctures — once arrayed side by side on a pantry shelf, they all begin to look alike!

DANDELION DOSAGES

Small doses are considered more restorative; large ones are more "heat-" or infection-clearing. When using dandelion in the form of medicine, dosage guidelines include:
- 1 cup of tea three or four times daily
- 30 drops of tincture in a bit of water three times daily
- 2 size "00" capsules three times daily

MEDICINAL TEA RECIPES

The tea recipes on the following pages can be used to treat, soothe, heal, or ease the symptoms of a variety of ailments and conditions. Ingredients are called for in parts, which will enable you to make as much of the recipe as is appropriate for your needs. Note that in the ingredients lists, the term "herb" refers to the aboveground portion of the plant, including the stem, leaf, and flower. And don't forget that the recipes can also be formu-lated as tinctures for potent yet portable remedies — see Making Herbal Tinctures.

Overcoming-Addiction Tea

This tea will lend strength and willpower when you've decided to give up caffeine, nicotine, alcohol, or even anything stronger. It strengthens the adrenal glands and cleanses and supports the nerves.

Infuse

    1 part skullcap *(Scutellaria lateriflora)* herb

    1 part oat straw *(Avena sativa)* herb

Decoct

    1 part dandelion root

    1 part ginseng *(Panax ginseng)* root, chopped or sliced

Allergy-Relief Tea

This formula soothes inflammation and helps the body be more resistant to allergens.

Infuse

    1 part nettle *(Urtica dioica)* leaf

    1 part mullein *(Verbascum thapsus)* leaf

Decoct

    1 part dandelion root

    1 part marsh mallow *(Althaea officinalis)* root

    ½ part licorice *(Glycyrrhiza glabra)* root

Improve-Anemia Tea

For those suffering from anemia, this tea is rich in minerals, especially iron, and helps build the blood.

Infuse

> 1 part dandelion leaf
> 1 part nettle *(Urtica dioica)* leaf
> 1 part watercress *(Nasturtium officinale)* leaf

Decoct

> 1 part yellow dock *(Rumex crispus)* root

Arthritis-Relief Tea

Ease your joints with this anti-inflammatory preparation. It also helps strengthen the immune system.

Infuse

> 1 part nettle *(Urtica dioica)* leaf

Decoct

> 1 part dandelion root
> 1 part yucca *(Yucca glauca)* root
> 1 part devil's claw *(Harpagophytum procumbens)* tuber

Blood-Sugar StabiliTea

This tea helps stabilize blood sugar levels and can benefit those suffering from hypoglycemia as well as those suffering from diabetes.

Infuse

> 1 part blueberry *(Vaccinium myrtillus)* leaf
> ½ part fennel *(Foeniculum vulgare)* seed
> 1 part fenugreek *(Trigonella foenum-graecum)* seed

Decoct

> 1 part dandelion root

Freshen-Bad-Breath Tea

Sweeten your breath with these mouth-freshening herbs!

Infuse

> 1 part dandelion leaf
> 1 part peppermint *(Mentha x piperita)* leaf
> ½ part cardamom *(Eletteria cardamomum)* seeds, crushed

Decoct

> 1 part cinnamon *(Cinnamomum zeylanicum)* chips

I'm-Sick-of-Cellulite Tea

Help your body metabolize fats and improve elimination of wastes with these cleansing herbs.

Infuse

> 1 part dandelion leaf
>
> 1 part nettle *(Urtica dioica)* leaf

Decoct

> 1 part dandelion root
>
> 1 part burdock *(Arctium lappa)* root

Children's Feel-Better Tea

These herbs can help the body fight infection and comfort the ailments of childhood, including colds, measles, mumps, and chickenpox.

Infuse

> 1 part lemon balm *(Melissa officinalis)* herb
>
> 1 part anise *(Pimpinella anisum)* seed
>
> 1 part peppermint *(Mentha piperita)* leaf

Decoct

> 1 part dandelion root
>
> 1 part echinacea *(Echinacea purpurea)* root

Lower-Cholesterol Tea

This tea blend helps the body gradually break down cholesterol and aids in its elimination.

Infuse

> 1 part hawthorn *(Crataegus oxycantha)* leaf, flower, or berry

Decoct

> 1 part dandelion root
>
> 1 part burdock *(Arctium lappa)* root
>
> 1 part ginger *(Zingiber officinale)* root

Clear-Skin Tea

By supporting the organs of elimination — the liver, kidneys, and colon — these herbs encourage clearer skin, especially for those suffering from acne, psoriasis, or eczema.

Decoct

> 1 part dandelion root
>
> 1 part burdock *(Arctium lappa)* root
>
> 1 part yellow dock *(Rumex crispus)* root
>
> 1 part Oregon grape *(Mahonia repens)* root

Alleviate-Depression Tea

Liver-cleansing, nerve-nourishing, and mood-elevating — consider these herbs when dealing with depression.

Infuse

> 1 part St.-John's-wort *(Hypericum perforatum)* herb
>
> 1 part oat straw *(Avena sativa)* herb
>
> 1 part lemon balm *(Melissa officinalis)* herb

Decoct

> 1 part dandelion root

Decongestion Tea

This tea helps the body to clear phlegm and open the lungs and sinuses.

Infuse

> 1 part dandelion leaf
>
> 1 part nettle *(Urtica dioica)* herb
>
> 1 part thyme *(Thymus vulgaris)* herb

Decoct

> 1 part dandelion root

Digestive Tea

When in need, reach for this multipurpose formula. It can aid in the digestion of fats, prevent gas, and soothe a stomachache.

Infuse

> 1 part dandelion leaf
> 1 part peppermint *(Mentha x piperita)* leaf
> ½ part fennel *(Foeniculum vulgare)* seed

Decoct

> 1 part dandelion root

Edema Tea

This tea helps the kidneys eliminate excess fluid from the body.

Infuse

> 1 part dandelion leaf
> 1 part nettles *(Urtica dioica)* leaf
> 1 part uva-ursi *(Arctostaphylos uva-ursi)* herb
> 1 part cornsilk *(Zea mays)* stigma

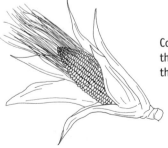

Cornsilk is the long, threadlike fibers found on the inside of the husk.

Increase Energy Tea

Try this tea instead of coffee in the morning. It's nourishing and mildly stimulating without the drawbacks of addiction and the jitters.

Infuse

> 1 part dandelion leaf
>
> 1 part yerba maté *(Ilex paraguariensis)* leaf
>
> 1 part nettle *(Urtica dioica)* leaf

Decoct

> 1 part dandelion root

Fasting Tea

When you're fasting, drinking this tea will provide minerals, improve your energy, and freshen your breath as well as help cleanse metabolic wastes.

Infuse

> 1 part nettle *(Urtica dioica)* leaf
>
> 1 part peppermint *(Mentha x piperita)* leaf
>
> 1 part fennel *(Foeniculum vulgare)* seed

Decoct

> 1 part dandelion root

Headache Tea

This tea not only helps to relieve pain and stress but also helps reduce inflammation.

Infuse

> 1 part chamomile *(Matricaria recutita)* flower
> 1 part peppermint *(Mentha x piperita)* leaf

Decoct

> 1 part dandelion root
> 1 part white willow *(Salix alba)* bark

Improve-Jaundice Tea

By improving liver function, these herbs help improve jaundice.

Decoct

> 1 part dandelion root
> 1 part burdock *(Arctium lappa)* root
> 1 part Oregon grape *(Mahonia repens)* root
> 1 part yellow dock *(Rumex crispus)* root
> ½ part turmeric *(Curcuma longa)* powder or chopped root

Menopause-Relief Tea

These cool and calming herbs support your hormones, build the blood, and help the liver break down excessive hormones.

Infuse

> 1 part vitex *(Vitex agnus-castus)* berry

Decoct

> 1 part dandelion root
>
> 1 part black cohosh *(Cimicifuga racemosa)* root
>
> 1 part dong quai *(Angelica sinensis)* root

Menstrual-Relief Tea

Rich in minerals, this blood-building tea improves liver function so that hormones can be metabolized and reduces stagnation in the breasts and reproductive system.

Infuse

> 1 part dandelion leaf
>
> 1 part nettle *(Urtica dioica)* leaf
>
> 1 part raspberry *(Rubus idaeus)* leaf

Decoct

> 1 part dandelion root
>
> 1 part dong quai *(Angelica sinensis)* root

Mineral-Rich Tea

This herbal blend provides a wide variety of minerals. It's exceptionally nourishing for the bones, teeth, hair, and nails.

Infuse
- 1 part dandelion leaf
- 1 part nettle *(Urtica dioica)* leaf
- 1 part horsetail *(Equisetum arvense)* herb
- 1 part oat straw *(Avena sativa)* herb

Nursing-Mother's Tea

This tea works to increase milk production and improve its nutritional quality.

Infuse
- 1 part dandelion leaf
- 1 part nettle *(Urtica dioica)* leaf
- ½ part fennel *(Foeniculum vulgare)* seed, crushed

Decoct
- 1 part marsh mallow *(Althaea officinalis)* root

Pregnancy Tea

When you're pregnant, drink this nutritive tonic to tonify the uterus and help ease morning sickness.

Infuse

> 1 part dandelion leaf
>
> 1 part red raspberry *(Rubus idaeus)* leaf
>
> 1 part nettle *(Urtica dioica)* leaf

Decoct

> ½ part ginger *(Zingiber officinale)* root

Prostate Protection Tea

This tea improves circulation to the genitourinary system and reduces prostate inflammation.

Infuse

> 1 part dandelion leaf
>
> 1 part nettle *(Urtica dioica)* leaf

Decoct

> 1 part dandelion root
>
> 1 part saw palmetto *(Serenoa serrulata)* berry
>
> 1 part marsh mallow *(Althaea officinalis)* root

....

Sleep-Better Tea

Sleep better with these nerve-nourishing, calming herbs.

Infuse

    1 part dandelion leaf

    1 part linden *(Tilia platyphyllos)* flower

    1 part passion flower *(Passiflora incarnata)* herb

Decoct

    1 part kava-kava *(Piper methysticum)* root

....

Postsurgery/Recovery Tea

This is an excellent blend for cleansing drug residue out of the body and building strength and energy.

Infuse

    1 part dandelion leaf

    1 part nettle *(Urtica dioica)* leaf

Decoct

    1 part dandelion root

    ½ part licorice *(Glycyrrhiza glabra)* root

    1 part Siberian ginseng *(Eleutheroccus senticosus)* root

Swollen-Glands Tea

Try this blend for mumps, tonsillitis, and any glandular swelling. It works to improve lymphatic function.

Infuse

> 1 part dandelion leaf
> 1 part cleavers *(Galium aparine)* herb

Decoct

> 1 part dandelion root
> 1 part echinacea *(Echinacea purpurea)* root

Urinary-Tract-Infection Tea

This tea is diuretic and soothing to inflammation in the urinary tract; it also helps to fight infection.

Infuse

> 1 part dandelion leaf
> 1 part uva-ursi *(Arctostaphylos uva-ursi)* herb
> 1 part cornsilk *(Zea mays)* stigmas
> 1 part buchu *(Barosma betulina)* leaf

Decoct

> 1 part marsh mallow *(Althaea officinalis)* root

Improve-Vision Tea

Improve your vision with the eye-nourishing herbs in this blend. They provide beta-carotene and lutein and increase circulation to the eyes.

Infuse

1 part dandelion leaf
1 part dandelion flower
½ part bilberry *(Vaccinium myrtillus)* powder
1 part eyebright *(Euphrasia officinalis)* herb

Decoct

1 part dandelion root

Vitamin C–Rich Tea

These vitamin C–rich herbs are also high in flavonoids, which help improve the body's assimilation of that nutrient.

Infuse

1 part dandelion leaf
1 part rose *(Rosa canina)* hip
1 part hibiscus *(Hibiscus rosa-sinensis)* flower
1 part raspberry *(Rubus idaeus)* leaf

The-Weather-Is-Cold-and-I-Have-to-Be-Outside Tea

Warm yourself with the circulation-supporting herbs in this blend.

Decoct

>   1 part roasted dandelion root
>   1 part ginger *(Zingiber officinale)* root
>   1 part cinnamon *(Cinnamomum zeylanicum)* bark
>   ½ part licorice *(Glycyrrhiza glabra)* root
>   ½ part prickly ash *(Zanthoxylum americanum)* bark

Weight-Loss Tea

Help the body metabolize fat, eliminate excess water, remain ener-getic, and control its appetite with this blend.

Infuse

>   1 part dandelion leaf
>   1 part nettle *(Urtica dioica)* leaf
>   1 part yerba maté *(Ilex paraguariensis)* leaf
>   1 part hawthorn *(Crataegus oxycantha)* leaf, flower, and/or berry

Decoct

>   1 part dandelion root

MAKING JUICE

Dandelion leaves and roots can be put through a juicer to make a valuable tonic that helps counteract hyperacidity and normalizes the alkalinity of the system. It is rich in calcium, iron, magnesium, potassium, and sodium. The juice combines well with carrots and is used therapeutically for bone, spinal, and dental weakness. Take 1 to 6 tablespoons daily of this supreme nutritive tonic.

....

Dandelion Juice

Two cups of leaves will make approximately ½ cup of juice.

Fresh dandelion leaves (and/or roots)

Cut or tear the leaves into small pieces. Run through a juicer. Store in the refrigerator.

....

Juice Benefits for Specific Ailments

People with arthritis should take ½ cup of dandelion juice morning and evening on an empty stomach. The effectiveness of the juice is enhanced with a small amount of watercress juice. The juice is also recommended in treatment of gout, obesity, hypertension, arteriosclerosis, Bright's disease, kidney stones, herpes, and night blindness (for this, make the juice from the flowers). As discussed in *Heinerman's Encyclopedia of Healing Juices,* S. Niedermeir, a German doctor, experimented with dandelion juice and found that it improved the eye disorders retinitis pigmentosa (atrophy of the inner layers of the eye's filtering system) and nyctalopeia (also known as night blindness).

There is also some indication that dandelion juice may benefit tuberculosis: Its high beta-carotene content as well as its rich reserves of calcium and potassium salts help to "strip" the bacteria from mucosal tissue in the lungs. Also, the lutein helps to disinfect the lungs, making it difficult for bacteria to adhere to them.

MAKING CAPSULES

You can also treat dandelion leaves and roots to go into capsules. (Pull-apart capsules are available from most health-food stores and herb shops.) Powder the dried herb in a blender, a handful at a time, fill both halves of the empty capsules, and fit the halves together. Two dandelion capsules may be taken up to three times a day, as needed, for medicinal purposes.

DANDELION AS A HOMEOPATHIC REMEDY

The homeopathic dandelion remedy *Taraxacum,* available in most health-food stores and herb shops, is made from an alcohol tincture of the entire plant before the flower opens. As it is in herbology, homeopathic usage of dandelion is for treating liver and digestive disorders. It is a remedy for ague, appetite loss, biliousness, debility, diabetes, flatulence (a feeling of bubbles in the bowels), gallstones, jaundice, liver, neuralgia, night sweats, rheumatism, a bitter taste in the mouth, an irritated tongue whose tissue is left raw and sore, and typhoid fever. It is used to treat frequent urination with difficulty in the passing of the urine and also extreme thirst. *Taraxacum* is usually given in a 1x or 3x potency.

SYRUPS

Syrups can be a delicious way to obtain the health and nutritional benefits of dandelions, and can be used daily or on occasion. They are an excellent method for persuading children to take herbal remedies. Syrups contain a lot of sugar, however, so use them in moderation.

....

Dandelion Spring Tonic Syrup

This spring tonic should be made with a variety of the spring herbs that grow wild in your area, such as dandelion leaves and roots, nettles, chickweed, and plantain. Because this recipe calls for brandy, it should not be used by pregnant women or alcohol-intolerant persons.

> Several handfuls of wild spring herbs (enough so the water just covers)
> 4 cups water
> 1 cup fruit juice concentrate
> ½ cup brandy

1. Chop the herbs and place in a pot. Add the water (which should be enough to just cover them). Bring to a boil, reduce heat, and simmer until the liquid is reduced by half and is thick and dark colored. Strain, reserving the liquid. You should have approximately 1 pint.

2. Mix in the fruit juice concentrate and the brandy. Pour into a glass container and store in the refrigerator. This syrup will keep for several months.

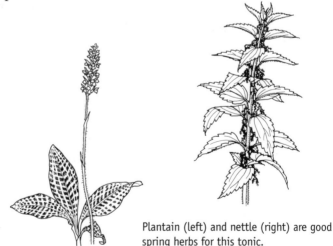

Plantain (left) and nettle (right) are good spring herbs for this tonic.

Dandelion Flower Syrup

Use as a spread on bread and butter as you would honey.

> 2 very large handfuls of dandelion flowers
> 1 quart cold water
> 5 cups unrefined sugar
> ½ lemon, including peel

1. Place the dandelions in the water and bring to a boil. Remove from heat, cover, and allow to steep overnight.

2. The next day, strain and press the flowers to remove the liquid. Add the sugar and the lemon, peel and all. Bring to a boil, reduce heat, and simmer until the mixture is of a syrup consistency.

3. Remove the lemon and pour the syrup into a glass container. Store in the refrigerator.

DELICIOUS DANDELION BEVERAGES

In addition to medicinal teas, dandelions can provide a multitude of healthful, pleasant-tasting, nutrient-rich beverages. Drinking dandelions can even alleviate some of the harmful effects of drinking too much coffee. Dandelions can also be enjoyed in the traditional alcoholic forms of wine and beer, and as a cordial.

Dandelion Coffee

One of my favorite beverages is a dandelion "coffee" made from the dried and roasted roots. This drink tastes rich and earthy, similar to coffee, but without the caffeine. It is nonaddictive and much kinder to the stomach. Dandelion roots tend to be more bitter in summer and fall and sweeter in spring.

GIVING UP COFFEE FOR GOOD

Some people use the rich brew made from dandelion roots to extend their coffee and thus decrease the amount of caffeine they are ingesting. To give up coffee, gradually use less coffee and more dandelion root. By doing this over time, you can bypass the caffeine-withdrawal headache. Drinking dandelion root coffee helps to diminish the craving for coffee flavor, as it has such a rich, earthy, roasted taste. Also consider dosages of the Overcoming-Addiction Tea (page 46), which can help strengthen both your willpower and your nerves.

To prepare the roots: Dig the roots (20 should give you enough for a small supply) in the fall and wash well, using a vegetable brush to scrub them. Slice the roots lengthwise and allow them to dry in a warm place for two weeks.

To roast the roots: When dry, roast them for 4 hours in an oven heated to 200°F (93°C). An alternative is to roast the dried, sliced roots in a cast-iron skillet, stirring constantly until they are dark brown. Cool completely before storing in a glass jar. Roasting dandelion roots releases aromatic compounds and converts the starch inulin into fructose, sweetening their taste.

*Dandelions are
Nature's way of
giving dignity to
weeds.*

*— MARVIN,
CARTOON CHARACTER*

To brew: Simmer 1 heaping teaspoon of the root in a cup of water, covered, for 10 minutes, then strain. The resulting dark, rich beverage will help you feel warmer. If you wish you can also use the roasted roots as a coffee substitute by percolating or using the drip method.

To enjoy: You can drink this as you would coffee with cream and sugar or with honey and milk.

Warming Winter Spice Tea

Slowly heat 4 cups of spring water in a pot. Put the following ingredients into a mortar and with a pestle crush the herbs slightly. Or put them into a blender and turn it on briefly, just enough to release some of the aromas.

Decoct

    2 parts roasted dandelion root

    ½ part cinnamon bark

    ½ part dried gingerroot

    ½ part decorticated (hulled) cardamom seeds

    ½ part star anise

    Honey to taste

    Milk or nondairy substitute to taste (optional)

Dandelion Mocktail

    100 small dandelion leaves, washed

    1½ cups tomato juice

    2 tablespoons Worcestershire sauce

    A dash of Tabasco sauce

    2 to 3 stalks of celery

Blend together all the ingredients. Garnish with a celery stalk. Yield: 2 to 3 servings

Dandelion Wine

Dandelion wine, believed to be of Celtic origin, is regarded as one of the fine country wines of Europe. In the late 1800s and early 1900s, it was not proper for ladies to drink alcohol; however, dandelion flower wine was considered so therapeutic to the kidneys and digestive system that it was deemed medicinal even for the ladies.

3 quarts dandelion blossoms

1 gallon water

2 oranges, with peel

1 lemon, with peel

3 pounds sugar

1 ounce fresh yeast

1 pound raisins

1. Collect the blossoms when they are fully open on a sunny day. Remove any green parts; they will impair the fermentation.

2. Bring the water to a boil and pour it over the flowers in a large pot. Cover and let steep for 3 days.

3. Peel and juice the oranges and the lemon, saving the peels and reserving the liquid.

4. Add the orange and lemon peel to the flower-water mixture and bring to a boil. Remove from heat, strain out the solids, then add the sugar, stirring until it is dissolved. Allow to cool.

5. Add the orange and lemon juice, yeast, and raisins to the liquid. Put everything into a crock with a loose lid (so gas can escape) to ferment.

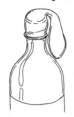

A deflated balloon will help you moniter fermentation.

6. When the mixture has stopped bubbling (2 days to a week), fermentation is complete. Strain the liquid through several layers of cheesecloth and transfer to sterilized bottles. Slip a deflated balloon over the top of each bottle to moniter for further fermentation. When the balloon remains deflated for 24 hours, fementation is complete. Cork the bottles and store in a cool, dark place for at least 6 months before drinking.

Dandelion Beer

During Victorian times in England, dandelion stout was offered for sale.

> 1 quart fresh dandelion leaves (from young
> unflowered plants) with some roots
> 1 gallon plus ¾ cup of spring water
> Dandelion blossoms (sepals removed)
> 1½ cups brown or unrefined sugar
> 1 tablespoon cream of tartar
> Juice of ½ lemon
> 1 tablespoon granulated bread yeast (be sure
> it has no preservatives)

1. Place the dandelion leaves and roots in a large pot, add 1 gallon of water, and bring to a boil. Reduce heat, cover, and simmer for 30 minutes. Remove from heat and allow to cool.

2. In a small bowl, mix the yeast with ¾ cup of the water and 1 tablespoon of the sugar. Cover and place in a warm area for 10 minutes, until it starts to foam. Pour into a large bowl with the dandelion water and add the rest of the sugar, the cream of tartar, and the lemon juice. Let sit for 30 minutes, then stir thoroughly.

3. Cover the bowl and keep at 65 to 70°F (18 to 21°C) for 12 to 24 hours, stirring occasionally with a wooden spoon until the mixture starts fizzing.

4. Transfer the liquid to sterilized bottles and leave them out at room temperature for 3 hours, then refrigerate for 3 days. The beer will keep for 1 week. (If you have more than you can drink in that amount of time, invite some friends over to share this tasty brew!)

Dandelion Fizz

5 cups dandelion flowers, washed, stems removed
4½ quarts water
4 cups sugar
2 lemons (sliced, with peel)

1. Bring the water to a boil. Place the dandelions in a crock and pour the boiling water over them. Cover and allow to stand for 12 hours.

2. Strain the dandelion water through several layers of cheesecloth into a large pot. Add the sugar and lemon. Heat gently to allow the sugar to dissolve, but not so much that the mixture boils, then remove from heat.

3. Strain the liquid into sterilized bottles and allow to cool. Apply caps and store in a cool, dry place. After 3 to 4 weeks, the fizz will be ready to drink and should be stored in the refrigerator. It will keep for 3 to 4 months.

Dandelion Cordial

3 cups dandelion flowers
⅔ cup honey
Rind of ½ lemon
1 quart vodka

1. Remove the dandelion petals from the green portions, but don't wash them; compost the green part.

2. Mix together the dandelion petals, the honey, the lemon rind, and the vodka and pour into a widemouth jar. Cap tightly and store in a cool, dry place for 2 weeks, shaking the jar every day.

3. Strain the ingredients through a fine strainer or several layers of cheesecloth. Discard the solids and rebottle the liquid. Drink it by itself or with a slice of lemon.

TOPICAL MEDICINAL USES

Generally speaking, dandelion leaves are rich in chlorophyll, which speeds wound healing and helps prevent infection. The roots are cooling and can be used to help draw out and deter infections. Together, they could be prescribed for a number of specific health concerns.

Skin Irritations

Dandelion sap can be applied topically to bee stings, blisters, calluses, corns, and warts. The bitter white juice is most potent when the plant is in flower, in the spring or summer — sap taken from plants in the fall or winter will not be as effective. Just break open the stem or root and apply the sap to the area. Do this twice a day for five days.

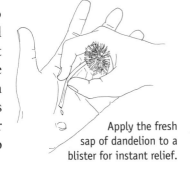

Apply the fresh sap of dandelion to a blister for instant relief.

Breast Health

Dandelion flower massage oil (see recipe on page 72) is recommended for breast massage. It helps to release the negative emotions stored in the breast tissue and improves lymphatic movement. It is very helpful for those prone to breast cysts and lumps, and is a way of nurturing and giving positive attention to the breasts. You can also use a poultice of the fresh grated roots or leaves to treat breast concerns such as cancer, cysts, and mastitis.

Fighting Infections

Use dandelion leaf as a bath herb to discourage yeast infections. For women who suffer from such infections, add a couple of handfuls of the leaves to the bathwater. Run the water hot. Or place the leaves in a discarded sock and secure it with a hair tie to make cleanup easier — you'll still get the medicinal benefits in the tub. Dandelion leaf tea is also used as a wash in treating fungal infections.

Dandelion Massage Oil

The proportion of dandelion to olive oil isn't an important factor in making this massage oil. Simply keep in mind that the more blossoms you use, the more potent the oil. This is an excellent remedy to use for breast massage (see Breast Health on page 71) as well as to help skin heal.

Dandelion blossoms
Dandelion root
Extra-virgin olive oil

1. Collect blossoms on a sunny dry day in the morning, after the dew has evaporated. Spread them on a screen and set them to dry in a cool, dry, shady, well-ventilated area for 2 to 3 days.
2. The day before you plan to make the oil, gather some dandelion roots. Wash them well and allow to dry overnight.
3. Chop up the dried roots. Place the blossoms and the chopped roots in a small glass jar. Cover with olive oil. Stir with a nonmetal utensil (such as a wooden chopstick) to force out any air bubbles, then top off with more oil. Seal and store in a cool, dry location at room temperature for 6 weeks.
4. Strain the infused oil through several layers of cheesecloth. Discard the spent herb and rebottle and label the liquid. Refrigerated, the oil will keep for 3 to 4 months.

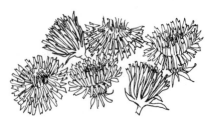

Dandelion Flower Essence

Dandelion flower essence, available from natural food stores and herb shops, helps promote relaxation and facilitates the release of negative emotions that are bound up in muscles, especially in the back, neck, and shoulders. It's an excellent flower essence to use when having bodywork, such as massage, done. It is also an excellent remedy for those who use their bodies a lot, such as massage therapists and athletes.

Dandelion flower essence also benefits those of us who over-structure our lives and find ourselves too busy to relax. It improves body-mind communication in tense people. It helps us to let go of fear and have more trust in our ability to cope with life. By relaxing the physical body, it fosters spiritual openness and yet enables us to listen to and hear the messages of our body. It is used for people dealing with cancer or muscular degeneration, nervous people, and those with poor posture. It is also good for people who have a fear of being touched.

COSMETIC USES

Dandelion also has potential for cosmetic use. Dandelion is rich in emollients, which makes it useful in treating dry, sallow, and mature skins. Dandelion root tea is considered toning, meaning it helps to invigorate the skin and brings out more beauty, and it can help to revitalize sallow skin. You can also blend the leaves with a bit of water and apply to the face as a mask to brighten sallow skin. The leaves can also be used in facial steams and herbal baths (see page 74) to soothe and cleanse the skin.

Age Spots

Age spots, also known as brown spots or liver spots, usually appear on the backs of the hands and are caused by the cumulative effects of sunlight or chronic bruising of the skin. Fresh dandelion sap, collected when the plant is in bloom in the spring or summer, can be applied directly to age spots to lighten them.

Herbal Bath

Adding dandelion to the bath helps remedy eczema and dry, oily, or itchy skin. It is also used as a bath herb for those who wish to lose weight.

1 pint of water

2 heaping teaspoons dried dandelion herb

To make and use:

1. Bring the water to a boil, then pour over the dandelion. Cover and let steep for 30 minutes.

2. Strain the infused tea and compost the spent herb. Add the tea to a full, warm bath, then get in for a soak!

Facial Steam

This gentle treatment will leave you with a fresh, radiant complexion.

1 pint water

2 heaping teaspoons dried dandelion leaves

To make and use:

1. Bring the water to a boil. Remove from heat, stir in the dandelion leaves, and set the hot pot on a table or countertop.

2. Sitting down at a comfortable height, position your head so that your face is about 10 inches away from the surface of the

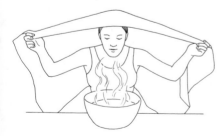

pot. Drape a towel over the pot and your head to contain the steam, and inhale the vapors and steam your facial skin for 5 minutes.

3. Rinse with a cold water splash and pat dry.

Dandelion Flower Water

In the 1800s, European women used dandelion flower water to lighten freckles, age spots, and small moles, and it's still used today to promote healthy clear skin and prevent and treat blemishes.

1 cup freshly gathered, opened dandelion flowers
1½ cups spring water

To make:
1. Put the flowers and water in a pan and bring to a boil. Cover and simmer for 30 minutes.
2. Strain, squeezing the excess liquid out of the flowers, and store in a glass bottle in the refrigerator.
To use:
Apply to face with a cotton ball.

Dandelion Skin Oil

This facial oil helps to soften the skin. It also helps to disperse the congestion that contributes to breakouts.

4 fresh, medium-size dandelion leaves
5 tablespoons castor oil

To make:
1. Wash, dry, and chop the dandelion leaves. Place them in a small pan with the castor oil and bring to a boil. Simmer for 10 minutes, then remove from heat. Cover and allow to steep for 3 hours.
2. Strain the infused oil into a glass jar, and discard the spent herb. Store in the refrigerator.
To use:
Apply to skin blemishes as necessary, using a clean cotton cloth or a cotton ball.

Dandelion Moisturizing Milk

This is both cleansing and moisturizing. It's excellent for improving sallow complexions.

¼ pint spring water

3 tablespoons elder flowers

2 tablespoons dandelion leaves

½ cup milk

To make:

1. Bring the water to a boil. Pour over the elder flowers and dandelion leaves, stir, cover, and let steep for 12 hours.

2. Add the milk, mix well, and let steep another 2 hours. Strain into a glass container and store in the refrigerator.

To use:

Apply gently to face with a cotton ball.

Facial Wash

A large handful of fresh-picked dandelion blossoms

1 pint water

To make:

1. Bring the water to a boil, then pour over the blossoms. Cover and let steep for 1 hour.

2. Strain to separate the flowers from the liquid.

To use:

1. Apply the flowers (with some of the liquid) to the face and lie down for 10 minutes.

2. Use the remaining liquid to rinse your face — no need to finish with water.

OTHER PRACTICAL USES

Dandelion has served humanity in diverse ways. Not only can it feed, nourish, and enhance beauty, it can bring color and comfort into our lives.

- As a dye plant, dandelion root turns wool magenta when alum is used as a mordant, purple when tin and vinegar are used, and yellow when no mordant (fixative) is added. The flowers yield a yellow dye.
- During World War II, the latex sap from the root of the Russian dandelion *(Taraxacum koksaghyz),* which is said to yield four times the latex of other species, was used to make rubber.
- When dandelions are dried and mixed with potpourri, they add bulk and color (though not much aroma).
- There are reports of dandelion leaves being dried and used as a smoking mixture to help asthma. The leaves are combined with equal parts of mullein and rosemary and smoked very slowly in a waterpipe.

Dandelion Dye

To make a light yellow dye for wool from the roots, no mordant is required.

> 1 gallon roots, chopped
> 1½ gallons water

To make and use:

1. Place the roots in a large pot and fill with the water. Allow to soak overnight.

2. Bring the mixture to a boil, reduce heat, and simmer for 1 hour. Then strain and discard the spent roots.

3. Add enough cold water to make a total of 2 gallons of liquid. Bring to a boil, add wet wool, reduce heat, and simmer for 1 hour.

4. Rinse and dry the wool.

6

COOKING WITH DANDELIONS

Dandelions provide a multitude of culinary possibilities. The young leaves are most commonly used and should be gathered before the flower stalk achieves full height and before the flowers have yet formed. Try adding them raw to salads or in place of lettuce on sandwiches. Add them to cooked dishes such as soups, rice dishes, stir-fries, and omelets. Try juicing the fresh leaves and roots with carrots and spinach for a nutrient-rich beverage. You can substitute dandelion greens in most recipes that call for spinach.

Young dandelion flowers have a sweet, honeylike flavor; they get a bit more bitter as they age. Pick the flowers immediately before using so that they won't close up. Keep in mind that the green sepals attached to the flowers can be somewhat tart — great for some recipes, undesirable for others.

Consider how much time has passed since produce from the supermarket may have been picked, and from how many miles away it was transported. Now think about how wonderful it is to use something free, fresh, and local!

> ## Tip
>
> The best-tasting leaves are usually gathered from the center of plants growing in shady areas.

Preparing the Leaves

Old herbals report that it is better to wash and shred the leaves by hand rather than cutting them with a knife. When the leaves are cut, cells are torn and that causes the release of an enzyme called ascorbic acid oxidase, which depletes vitamin C. It is always best to shred the leaves right before they are going to be used to help conserve nutrients.

> ## Measuring It Out
>
> One pound of fresh greens equals 2 quarts, and when cooked yields 1½ to 2 cups of cooked greens.

Cooking the Leaves

You can eat young leaves raw, but as they get older they are more palatable cooked. The French soak the leaves in salt water for half an hour to remove bitterness; however, this does somewhat decrease the nutritional value. Even after the leaves become bitter, I still add them to certain dishes, as a little bitterness stimulates digestive secretions. However, you can minimize the sharp taste by cooking first in two changes of salted water or by adding a small amount of vinegar to the finished dish. After the first frost, the bitterness is dispersed and the leaves can easily be enjoyed again.

The chlorophyll content of dandelion leaves is sensitive to acids. When the leaves are cooked, the chlorophyll reacts with natural acids in the cooking water. A reaction with the carotene pigments causes a brown compound called pheophytin to form. To prevent the chlorophyll from reacting with any acids, leave the lid off the pot when cooking so that the acids may evaporate, or steam the plant quickly so there is little time for a reaction to occur. One other method is to cook the plant in plenty of water so that the acids are diluted. If you do this, though, do what wise Italians suggest: Drink the leftover water, which is said to beautify appearance.

Boiling dandelions will deplete some of their nutritional value, so steaming and stir-frying are the best methods of cooking.

NUTRITIONAL AND HEALTHFUL CONSTITUENTS

Dandelion is considered one of the five most nutritious vegetables on earth. Popeye may have gotten strength from spinach, but dandelion has twice the vitamin B_1 of that vegetable and six times the iron and four times the B_2 of iceberg lettuce. It contains 40 percent more vitamin C than tomatoes, 20 percent more beta-carotene than carrots, and more calcium than milk. One hundred grams of dandelion leaves provides 14,000 IU of pro-vitamin A, whereas carrots provide 11,000. At only 45 calories per 100 grams, these generous greens are also a rich source of iron, manganese, and phosphorus. Choline, the member of the B complex that helps to prevent fat buildup in the liver, is also present.

As every health-conscious individual knows, good nutrition is the most important part of good health. As evidenced by the lengthy lists that follow, not only does dandelion contain most of the vitamins and minerals recommended for a healthy diet — the ones you'll see called out in the nutritional information posted on the label of any packaged food — but it's also packed with a dizzying range of enzymes, acids, sugars, and other substances that nourish the health and energy of your entire body and all of its systems.

"SEASON WITH DANDELION TO TASTE"

Dandelion greens are so good for you that you would do well to dry and powder them and place the powder in a salt shaker to be sprinkled on all your food as a nutritional supplement.

WHAT THE ROOT CONTAINS

CONSTITUENT	NATURE/BENEFIT
Asparagin	Acts as a natural diuretic.
Caffeic acid	Helps treat allergies due to its anti-inflammatory properties.
Calcium	Nourishes bones, teeth, and nerves.
Choline	Helps metabolize fats and aids nerve and brain transmissions.
Coumestrol	A phytoestrogenic substance.
Essential oil	Contains antimicrobial properties.
Fatty acids (myristic, palmitic, stearic, lauric)	Benefit the nervous system and aid fat metabolism and digestion.
Flavonoid glycosides (apigenin and luteolin)	Exhibit diuretic, antispasmodic, antioxidant, and hepatoprotective properties.
Flavonoids (lutein, flavoxanthin, violaxanthin)	Natural antioxidants.
Fructose	A fruit sugar.
Gallic acid	Tones tissues due to its astringent properties.
Hydroxyphenylacetic acid	Natural antioxidants.
Hydroxyphenylacetic gum	Soothes inflammation.
Hydroxyphenylacetic resin	Naturally antiseptic.
Inulin	Helps to keep blood sugar levels stable. The content is highest in autumn, up to 24 percent.
Iron	Builds the blood.
Lactupicrine (bitter principle)	Stimulates natural digestive secretions.
Levulin	Starch, most concentrated in spring roots.
Mucilage	Soothes irritation.
Pectin	A soluble fiber that may contribute to the plant's detoxifying abilities. In Russia, pectin is recommended to help the body detoxify from heavy metals and radioactivity.
Phenolic acids (including quinic acid and chlorogenic acid)	Known for their antimicrobial properties.
Phosphorus	Benefits the heart and brain.
Polysaccharides (glucans, mannans, inulin)	Stimulate the immune system and benefit white blood cell production.

(continued on next page)

WHAT THE ROOT CONTAINS (continued)

CONSTITUENT	NATURE/BENEFIT
Potassium	Supports the kidneys and heart; dandelions contain about three times the potassium of most other greens.
Tannin	Restores tissue tone.
Taraxacerin	A crystalline, bitter substance.
Taraxacin	A bitter amorphous principle (root and leaves).
Triterpenes	Include taraxol, taraxerol, taraxasterol, and amyrin, and may play a role in dandelion's liver- and bile-stimulating properties.
Zinc	Supports the immune system.

Note: Taraxacin and taraxacerin are both actually combinations of triterpenoids and sterols (sitosterin, stigmasterin, phytosterin). These steroids have a structure similar to bile.

WHAT THE LEAVES CONTAIN

CONSTITUENT	NATURE/BENEFIT
Boron	Necessary for calcium metabolism and bone health.
Calcium lactate mannite	Builds healthy bones and teeth and supports heart function.
Chlorophyll	Helps cleanse bile from the blood and improves blood quality; helps the body utilize oxygen, prevents infection, and speeds wound healing.
Choline	A component of lecithin that helps to improve memory, nourish the nervous system, and prevent fat buildup in the liver.
Coumarin	Improves blood circulation.
Eudesmannolide	Believed to play a part in dandelion's diuretic properties.
Fatty acids (linoleic and linolenic)	Help in prostaglandin production, aiding immune response and reducing inflammatory conditions.
Flavonoid glycosides (apigenin and luteolin)	Improve circulation.
Folic acid	Builds the blood and helps prevent birth defects.
Germacranolide	May play a part in dandelion's diuretic properties.
Inositol	Helps nourish the brain and nervous system.
Iron	Builds the blood.

WHAT THE LEAVES CONTAIN (continued)

CONSTITUENT	NATURE/BENEFIT
Lecithin	Helps fat metabolism and nourishes the brain, nervous system, and heart.
Nicotinic acid	Improves circulation and aids fat metabolism.
Potassium	Strengthens cardiovascular function.
Sesquiterpene lactones	Include lactucin, lactucopikrin, and taraxacoside; antispasmodic, sedative, and anti-inflammatory properties.
Silica	Helps to rebuild connective tissue and nourishes bones, hair, teeth, and nails.
Terpenoids	Act as nerve nutrients.
Vitamin A	Strengthens mucous membranes and helps prevent infection; 100 grams of leaves contain 14,000 IU of vitamin A (more than carrots!).
Vitamin B	Supports the nervous system.
Vitamin C	Improves immune function and is necessary for collagen production.
Vitamin D	For healthy skin and bones.

WHAT THE FLOWERS CONTAIN

CONSTITUENT	NATURE/BENEFIT
Carotenoids (taraxanthin, which is actually a mixture of lutein, flavoxanthin, violaxanthin, and chrysanthemaxanthin)	Strengthen the mucous membranes, boost the immune system, and are antioxidant (lutein is also especially beneficial for the eyes).
Lecithin	Nourishes the brain and nervous system and enhances fat metabolism.

WHAT THE SAP CONTAINS

CONSTITUENT	NATURE/BENEFIT
Ceryl alcohol, tartaric acid, glycerin, caoutchouc, ester of acetic acids	Have shown a mild effect against candida.

The inulin present in dandelion root is currently under study for its potential as an immunostimulant as well as an aid for the kidneys and pancreas. Inulin is digested not in the stomach but, rather, in the colon by naturally occurring bacteria. Inulin encourages the growth of healthy intestinal flora. In a study conducted in 1995 at Dunn Clinical Nutrition Center in Cambridge, England, eight subjects were given 15 grams of extra sugar daily for 15 days to feed unfriendly bacteria, such as *Candida albicans,* and then given 15 grams of inulin for 15 days (about the amount in 2 ounces of fresh dandelion root). Results showed that the inulin helped to increase beneficial bacteria in the colon called bifidobacteria, which led to the conclusion that inulin could help improve the microflora of the intestines.

NUTRITIONAL VALUE

100 grams (3.53 ounces) of raw dandelion leaves yields the following:

	RAW	COOKED
Calories	45	33
Protein	2.7 g	2 g
Fat	0.7 g	0.6 g
Carbohydrate	9.2 g	6.4 g
Fiber	1.6 g	1.3 g
Calcium	187 mg	140 mg
Phosphorus	66 mg	42 mg
Iron	3.1 mg	1.8 mg
Sodium	76 mg	44 mg
Magnesium	284 mg	71 mg
Potassium	397 mg	232 mg
Vitamin A	14,000 IU	11,700 IU
Thiamin	.19 mg	.13 mg
Riboflavin	.26 mg	.16 mg
Vitamin C	35 mg	18 mg
Water %	85.6	89.2

DANDELION RECIPES

If the multitude of healthful and nutritional constituents of dandelion blossoms, leaves, sap, and roots hasn't yet convinced you that dandelion is one of nature's best foods, try the following recipes!

Scrambled Eggs with Dandelion Greens

2 tablespoons vegetable oil

2 cups washed, chopped dandelion greens

6 organic eggs

2 tablespoons milk

¼ teaspoon salt

¼ teaspoon freshly ground black pepper

Makes 3–4 servings

1. In a skillet, heat the oil and add the dandelion greens. Stir gently until cooked, about 10 minutes.

2. In a separate bowl, mix the eggs, milk, salt, and pepper. Pour over the greens and stir-fry until the eggs are cooked, about 5 minutes.

3. Garnish with a slice of tomato and a sprig of parsley and serve immediately.

Dandelion Buds with Eggs

1 tablespoon vegetable oil

20 dandelion flower buds, unopened

4 organic eggs

1 tablespoon milk

Salt and freshly ground black pepper

Makes 2 servings

1. Heat the oil in a skillet over medium heat.

2. Add the flower buds and stir until they start opening.

3. Mix in the eggs and milk, stirring gently with a fork, for 5 minutes, or until cooked to your liking. Season with salt and pepper and serve with crisp toast.

Dandelion Florentine Breakfast

4 cups washed, chopped dandelion greens

3 tablespoons low-fat cream cheese

4 organic eggs

Salt and freshly ground black pepper

Makes 4 servings

1. In a nonstick skillet over medium heat, stir the dandelion greens and cream cheese for about 3 minutes.

2. Make four little "nests" in the greens and add an organic egg to each of the indentations.

3. Cover and cook until the eggs are done, about 5 minutes.

4. Serve with a slice of whole-grain toast, and top off with some salsa if you like!

Dandelion Flower Pancakes

1 cup whole wheat flour

½ cup unbleached white flour

¼ teaspoon salt

1½ teaspoons baking soda

1½ cups milk (rice, soy, almond, oat, or dairy)

1 egg

⅔ cup dandelion flowers (sepals removed)

2 tablespoons vegetable oil

Makes about 4–6 pancakes

1. In a medium bowl, mix together the flours, salt, and baking soda.

2. In a separate bowl, beat togther the milk and egg, then stir into the dry ingredients.

3. Add the flowers and stir.

4. Add the vegetable oil and drop the pancake batter by spoonfuls onto a greased skillet. When the edges just start to brown, flip and cook on the other side.

5. Serve with real maple syrup and butter.

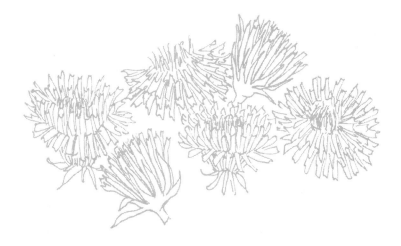

Dandelion Green Soup

1 medium onion, chopped fine

1 clove garlic, chopped

2 teaspoons curry powder

1 tablespoon olive oil

2 cups chopped potato

4 cups washed, chopped dandelion greens

4 cups water

½ teaspoon salt

Freshly ground black pepper

Tamari

Makes 6–8 servings

1. In a soup pot, sauté the onions, garlic, and curry powder in the olive oil, stirring constantly, until the onions are translucent.

2. Add the potatoes and dandelion greens and sauté briefly.

3. Add the water and cook until the potatoes are tender, about 30 minutes.

4. Cool for a short while, and then blend the soup pot ingredients in a blender. Return to the soup pot to reheat.

5. Season with salt, pepper, and tamari and serve hot.

Dandelions with Tofu

2 cups tofu

4 cups washed, chopped dandelion greens

½ teaspoon sea salt

Makes 4 servings

1. Mash the tofu and sauté in ¼ inch of boiling water, stirring constantly.

2. Add the dandelion greens and the salt, cover, and steam until tender, about 10 minutes. Serve hot garnished with fresh basil.

PREPARING DANDELION CROWNS

The crown, the portion between the leaf and the root, is white and tender and makes an excellent vegetable. Trim off the leaves and root (reserve for another recipe) and scrub the crown well to remove dirt. Boil in two changes of water. Season with a bit of butter, salt, and pepper. Crowns make an excellent addition to omelets, or you could also wash, chop, and add some to a salad. Another method of preparation is to steam until tender (about 4 minutes), then marinate in salad dressing and add to salads.

Dandelion crowns are the tender white part between the leaf and the root.

Dandelion Lasagna

3 cloves garlic

1 tablespoon parsley

1 tablespoon basil

1 tablespoon oregano

1 teaspoon fennel seed

1 tablespoon olive oil

6 cups washed, chopped dandelion greens

3 cups tomato sauce

6 ounces tomato paste

9 lasagna noodles

2 cups ricotta cheese

½ cup grated Parmesan cheese

1 cup grated mozzarella cheese

Makes 6 servings

1. Preheat the oven to 375°F (190°C).

2. Sauté the garlic, parsley, basil, oregano, and fennel in the olive oil, stirring until the garlic is cooked.

3. Add the dandelion greens, still stirring, and cook until they are wilted. Add the tomato sauce and paste and simmer for 2 hours, stirring occasionally.

4. Bring 2 quarts of water to a boil. Drop in the lasagna noodles and cook 5–7 minutes, until the pasta is tender. Drain and reserve.

5. In a greased baking dish place a layer of the noodles and cover with the sauce. Spread the cheeses evenly throughout. Cover with a layer of noodles. Layer again with sauce and cheeses. Cover with the remaining sauce.

6. Bake for 30 minutes, until cheese is nicely melted and sauce is bubbly. Serve immediately — French bread and a green salad make nice company!

Dandelion Green Quiche

You can also make this in a premade, 10-inch crust.

Crust

  ½ cup vegetable oil

  2 tablespoons milk

  ¾ cups unbleached white flour

  ¾ cup cornmeal

  1 tablespoon sage

  ½ teaspoon salt

  ¼ teaspoon pepper

1. Preheat the oven to 425°F (220°C).

2. Combine the liquids, then mix in the dry ingredients.

3. Press the dough into a 10-inch pie pan. Put in the oven and bake 5–7 minutes, until the edges are golden. Set aside.

Filling

  1 medium onion, chopped

  1 tablespoon vegetable oil

  1 cup grated cheese

  2½ cups washed, chopped dandelion greens

  2 eggs

  2 ounces cottage cheese

  Salt and freshly ground black pepper

Makes 6 servings

1. Lower the oven temperature to 350°F (180°C).

2. Lightly sauté the onion in the oil, then place in the prebaked pie shell. Add the grated cheese and the dandelion greens.

3. In a blender, whiz together the eggs, cottage cheese, and salt and pepper to taste. Pour over the greens in the pie shell.

4. Bake for 35 minutes, until the quiche is browned on top. Let stand a few minutes before serving.

Simple Dandelion Salad

3 cups young leaves from plants not yet bloomed, washed

10 flowers, washed, with sepals removed

Makes 4 servings

In a salad bowl, combine the leaves and flowers. Add your favorite salad dressing just before serving or make a dressing by mixing the following ingredients:

Simple Dressing

3 tablespoons olive oil

1 tablespoon tamari or soy sauce

1 teaspoon apple cider vinegar

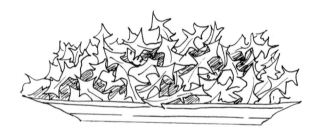

Served as a salad, mineral-rich dandelion greens have a pleasant taste and are deeply nourishing.

Dandelion Salad with Cottage Cheese and Pecans

2 cups washed, shredded dandelion greens

1 chopped tomato

1 tablespoon washed, chopped parsley

½ cup cottage cheese

¼ cup chopped toasted pecans (brown on a tray in the toaster oven for about 3 minutes)

2 tablespoons olive oil

2 teaspoons tamari or soy sauce

1 teaspoon lemon juice or apple cider vinegar

Makes 4 servings

In a salad bowl, arrange the greens, tomato, parsley, cottage cheese, and nuts. Toss with the oil, tamari, and lemon juice before serving.

Dandelion Spread

1 cup young washed, chopped dandelion leaves

½ cup cottage cheese

¼ cup toasted pecans

2 tablespoons salad dressing

Makes 4 servings

Mix all the ingredients in a blender and transfer to a pretty serving dish. Spread on crackers for a nice hors d'oeuvre.

Dandelion Flower Muffins

¼ cup vegetable oil

½ cup honey

1 egg

1 tablespoon baking powder

2 teaspoons cinnamon

½ teaspoon salt

2 cups milk (dairy, rice, soy, oat, or almond)

3 cups unbleached white flour

1 cup cornmeal

1 cup dandelion petals (without sepals)

½ cup washed, chopped dandelion leaves

Makes about 12 muffins

1. Preheat the oven to 350°F (180°C).

2. In a large bowl, mix together the oil and honey. Add the egg, baking powder, cinnamon, and salt, and mix thoroughly. Mix in the milk, flour, and cornmeal bit by bit, alternating ingredients.

3. Add the dandelion flowers and leaves and stir just enough to moisten all ingredients.

4. Spoon the batter into oiled muffin tins or paper wrappers and bake for 35 minutes, or until the tops are golden. Let cool for 10 minutes before attempting to remove the muffins from the tins. Enjoy as is or with butter or jam.

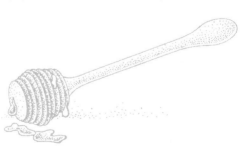

Dandelion Biscuits

1 cup whole wheat flour

¾ cup unbleached white flour

¼ teaspoon salt

2 teaspoons baking powder

2 tablespoons vegetable oil

½ cup dandelion flower petals (sepals removed)

¾ cup plain yogurt

Makes about 12–16 biscuits

1. Preheat the oven to 425°F (220°C).

2. Sift together the flours, salt, and baking powder. Add the oil, petals, and yogurt and stir for 3 minutes.

3. Turn the mixture onto a lightly floured board and roll it into a ball. With a rolling pin, roll to a thickness of ¼ inch. Cut with a 2-inch biscuit cutter or a jar lid of similar diameter.

4. Bake on a lightly oiled baking sheet for 12 minutes, until the biscuits are puffed up and golden. Enjoy with butter or gravy.

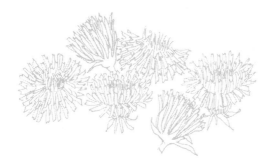

Dandelion Green Raita

1 cup washed and chopped dandelion greens

3 tablespoons plain yogurt

1 tablespoon olive oil

1 teaspoon lemon juice

½ teaspoon sea salt

Makes 2 servings

In a small bowl, combine all of the ingredients and toss gently. Serve with curries or other Indian food.

Dandelion Leaf Pesto

3 cloves garlic, chopped

½ cup olive oil

¼ cup shelled pine nuts

1½ cups washed, chopped fresh dandelion greens

¾ cup grated Romano cheese

Salt

Makes 2 servings

1. In a skillet over medium heat, slightly brown the garlic in the olive oil. Add the pine nuts and toast briefly. Stir in the dandelion greens, place the lid on the pan, and simmer for 10 minutes.
2. Remove the lid and add the cheese and salt to taste. Serve over rice, pasta, or potatoes, or on crackers.

Sweet and Sour Greens

4 cups young dandelion greens

2 tablespoons honey

¼ teaspoon powdered mustard

3 tablespoons apple cider vinegar

Salt and freshly ground black pepper

3 hard-boiled eggs, sliced

Makes 2 servings

1. Wash the greens well and pat dry.

2. Mix the honey, mustard, and vinegar with a bit of salt and pepper to taste. Pour over the dandelion greens and toss to coat. Garnish with the sliced eggs.

Greek Dandelion Horta

15 dandelion leaves

1 small onion, chopped

8 black olives

2 tablespoons olive oil

1 tablespoon apple cider vinegar

Salt and freshly ground black pepper

Makes 2 servings

1. Steam the dandelions and onion until both are tender.

2. Add the olives, oil, vinegar, and salt and pepper and mix gently. Serve as a side dish to accompany a festive Greek meal.

Creamed Dandelion Greens

6 cups washed, chopped dandelion greens

1½ tablespoons olive oil

1½ tablespoons unbleached white flour

1 cup milk

1½ cups grated sharp cheese

4 hard-boiled eggs, chopped

Makes 4 servings

1. Preheat the oven to 400°F (200°C).

2. Bring a pot of water to a boil. Add the greens and simmer for 10 minutes. Drain and set aside.

3. In a separate pan, heat the olive oil. Stir in the flour and slowly add the milk and cheese. Cook, stirring, until it thickens. Stir in the dandelions.

4. Remove from heat. Top with the eggs and bake in the oven for 15 minutes. Serve with a side of rice.

Dandelion Leaf Pizza

1 whole wheat pita pocket

½ cup tomato sauce

¾ cup chopped dandelion greens

2 slices mozzarella cheese

1 teaspoon chopped fresh basil

Makes 1 serving

1. Cover one side of the pita bread with the tomato sauce. Add the dandelion greens and top with cheese. Broil in a toaster oven until the cheese melts.

2. Remove from oven, top with basil, and serve immediately.

Dandelion Green Stir-Fry

½ cup walnuts

1 tablespoon olive oil

4 cloves garlic, minced

½ teaspoon grated gingerroot

4 cups washed, chopped dandelion greens

1 tablespoon tamari

Makes 2 servings

1. Toast the walnuts at 350°F for 10 minutes and set aside.

2. Heat the oil in a skillet and stir in the garlic and the ginger. Add the dandelion greens (still wet from being washed) and tamari. Cover and steam for 10 minutes, stirring occasionally. (Add a bit of water if it is too dry.) Top with the toasted walnuts before serving.

Dandelion Root Stir-Fry

3 tablespoons toasted sesame oil

1 cup sliced onion

4 cloves chopped garlic

2 cups washed, chopped early spring dandelion roots

2 tablespoons tamari

Makes 4 servings

1. Warm the oil in a skillet over medium heat. Add the onion and garlic and sauté for 3 minutes, or until the onions are transparent. Add the dandelion roots and cook 10 minutes or until tender, stirring occasionally.

2. Turn off heat and add the tamari. Serve immediately.

Dandelion Burgers

½ cup chopped onion

1 cup packed dandelion blossoms, stems and calyxes removed

½ cup unbleached white flour

2 tablespoons milk or milk substitute

½ teaspoon basil

½ teaspoon sage

½ teaspoon salt

3 tablespoons vegetable oil

Makes 3–4 burgers

1. Sauté the chopped onion.

2. Mix together all the ingredients including the sautéed onion and form into patties. Fry in a cast-iron pan coated with oil, about 3–5 minutes per side. Serve on a toasted bun or with a side of hash browns.

Cornmeal Dandelion Delights

1 egg

¼ cup finely grated Parmesan cheese

1 cup yellow cornmeal

¼ cup vegetable oil

20 dandelion blossoms

Makes 2–4 servings

1. Beat the egg and 1 teaspoon of water in a small bowl.

2. In a separate bowl, mix the cheese and cornmeal.

3. Heat the oil in a saucepan. Dip each flower into the egg mixture and then into the cornmeal, turning to coat. Drop the coated flowers into the heated oil, turning frequently, and sauté until browned. Drain on a paper towel. Serve as a side dish.

Dandelion Loaf

1 onion, chopped

1 stalk celery, chopped

2 tablespoons vegetable oil

1 teaspoon sage

1 cup dandelion flowers

1½ cups day-old bread, broken into 1-inch pieces

2 eggs

1 teaspoon salt

½ teaspoon freshly ground black pepper

1 tablespoon nutritional yeast

1 cup milk or milk substitute

Makes 6 servings

1. Preheat the oven to 350°F (180°C).

2. Sauté the onion and celery in the vegetable oil. Add the sage, the dandelion blossoms, bread, eggs, salt, pepper, and nutritional yeast. Mix well, then add the milk.

3. Pour into a greased baking dish and bake for 45 minutes, until the top has browned. Serve in slices with a vegetable side dish and salad.

Dandelion "Mushrooms"

15 dandelion blossoms, fresh picked and washed (leave moist)

½ cup unbleached white flour

¼ teaspoon sea salt

2 tablespoons vegetable oil or butter

Makes 2 servings

1. Coat the washed flowers with the flour and salt.

2. Heat the olive oil in a saucepan over medium. Add the coated flowers to the pan, turning to brown on all sides, about 2–3 minutes per side. Serve hot. This is excellent with a side dish of rice — it really tastes like mushrooms!

Dandelion Vinegar

Washed, chopped dandelion roots (enough to fill a glass container of your choice)

Apple cider vinegar

1. Place the chopped roots in a jar, packed well, and cover with apple cider vinegar. Cover and allow to steep for 6 weeks, shaking daily.

2. Strain out the roots and pour the vinegar into a clean container. Keep refrigerated and use in salad dressings or to flavor greens.

Dandelion Jelly

6 cups rinsed dandelion blossoms, stems removed

3 cups water

½ teaspoon orange extract

1 1-ounce box of pectin

4½ cups of sugar

Makes 4–6½-pint jars

1. In a large pot, place the dandelions in the water, bring to a boil, and simmer for 3 minutes. Remove from heat, drain, and discard (or compost) the plant material.

2. Add the orange extract and the box of pectin to 2⅔ cups of the liquid. Bring to a boil, then add the sugar. Return to boil, stirring constantly, until the sugar is dissolved. Remove from the heat.

3. Skim off any foam from the top. Pour the liquid into sterilized jars and seal. Store in a cool, dark place and refrigerate once opened.

Dandelion Pie

1 cup well-chopped dandelion leaves or dandelion blossoms removed from the calyx

⅔ cup honey

4 egg yolks

2 teaspoons grated (preferably organic) lemon peel

2 tablespoons unbleached white flour

1½ cups milk or milk alternative

½ cup sunflower seeds

1 unbaked frozen pie shell

Makes 8 servings

1. Preheat the oven to 350°F (180°C).

2. If you're using dandelion greens, cook them in ¼ cup water in a saucepan for 5 minutes, or until tender.

3. Mix together the honey, egg yolks, lemon peel, and flour. Slowly beat in the milk and cook over low heat, stirring until the custard thickens. Don't let the mixture scorch.

4. Blend the dandelions in a food processor. Add to the custard mixture and stir in the sunflower seeds.

5. Pour into the pie shell and bake for 20 minutes, until the top is browned.

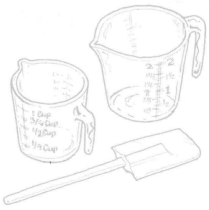

Dandelion Flower Cookies

½ cup vegetable oil

½ cup honey

2 eggs

1 teaspoon vanilla extract

1 cup unbleached white flour

1 cup oatmeal, powdered in the blender

½ cup dandelion petals, green portions removed

Makes 24 cookies

1. Preheat the oven to 350°F (180°C).

2. Blend the oil and honey. Mix in the eggs and vanilla; stir in the flour, oatmeal, and petals. Drop by the spoonful onto a lightly oiled baking sheet and bake for 12 minutes, until cookies begin to crisp.

FLOWER POPSICLES

Here's a quick summer treat children are sure to love. Fill popsicle molds with apple juice to which you've added the juice of a lime. Press a dandelion petal, removed from the calyx, into the center of each compartment. Freeze for at least 3 hours.

CONVERTING TO METRIC MEASUREMENTS

TEASPOONS TO MILLILITERS

¼ teaspoon = 1 ml

⅓ teaspoon = 2 ml

½ teaspoon = 2.5 ml

¾ teaspoon = 4 ml

1 teaspoon = 5 ml

TABLESPOONS TO MILLILITERS

¼ tablespoon = 4 ml

½ tablespoon = 8 ml

1 tablespoon = 15 ml

CUPS TO MILLILITERS

⅛ cup = 30 ml

¼ cup = 59 ml

⅓ cup = 79 ml

½ cup = 118 ml

⅔ cup = 150 ml

¾ cup = 180 ml

1 cup = 237 ml

2 cups = 473 ml = 1 pint

4 cups = 1 quart = 946 ml, or approximately 1 liter

4 quarts = 1 gallon = 4 liters

OUNCES TO GRAMS

¼ ounce = 7 g

⅓ ounce = 9.3 g

½ ounce = 14 g

1 ounce = 28 g

2 ounces = 56 g

3 ounces = 84 g

4 ounces = 112 g

6 ounces = 168 g

8 ounces = 224 g

16 ounces = 1 pound = 454 g

2.2 pounds = 1 kilogram

INCHES TO CENTIMETERS

1 inch = 2.5 cm

BIBLIOGRAPHY

Attenborough, David. *The Private Life of Plants.* Princeton, NJ: Princeton University Press, 1995.

Barash, Cathy Wilkinson. *Edible Flowers.* Golden, CO: Fulcrum Publishing, 1993.

Barnett, Robert. *Tonics.* New York: HarperCollins, 1997.

Bensky, Dan, Andrew Gamble, and Ted Kaptchuk. *Chinese Materia Medica.* Seattle: Eastland Press, 1986.

Bremness, Lesley. *The Complete Book of Herbs.* New York: Viking Studio Books, 1988.

Brown, Dr. O. Phelps. *The Complete Herbalist.* Van Nuys, CA: Newcastle Publishing, 1993.

Castleman, Michael. *The Healing Herbs.* Emmaus, PA: Rodale Press, 1991.

Chevallier, Andrew. *The Encyclopedia of Medicinal Plants.* New York: DK Publishing, 1996.

Cunningham, Donna. *Flower Remedies Handbook.* New York: Sterling Publishing Co., 1992.

D'Amelio, Frank. *The Botanical Practitioner.* Bellmore, NY: Holistic Publishing, 1982.

Dawson, Adele G. *Herbs, Partners in Life.* Rochester, VT: Healing Arts Press, 1991.

Dobelis, Inge N. *Magic and Medicine of Plants.* Pleasantville, NY: Reader's Digest Association, 1986.

Duke, James A., Ph.D. *The Green Pharmacy.* Emmaus, PA: Rodale Books, 1997.

Faber, K. "The Dandelion *Taraxacum officinale.*" *Il Pharmazie* 13:423–36, 1958.

Felter, Harvey Wicked, M.D., and John Uri Lloyd, Ph.D. *King's American Dispensatory.* Portland, OR: Eclectic Medical Publications, 1983.

Fielder, Mildred. *Plant Medicine and Folklore.* New York: Winchester Press, 1975.

Frawley, Dr. David and Dr. Vasant Lad. *The Yoga of Herbs.* Santa Fe, NM: Lotus Press, 1986.

Gail, Peter. *The Dandelion Celebration.* Cleveland, OH: Goosefoot Acres, 1994.

Grieve, Mrs. Maude. *A Modern Herbal*. New York: Dover Publications, 1971.

Harvey, Clare G., and Amanda Cochrane. *The Encyclopedia of Flower Remedies*. San Francisco: Thorson's, 1995.

Heinerman, John. *Heinerman's Encyclopedia of Healing Herbs and Spices*. West Nyack, NY: Parker Publishing, 1996.

———. *Heinerman's Encyclopedia of Healing Juices*. Englewood Cliffs, NJ: Prentice Hall, 1994.

———. *Scientific Validation of Herbal Medicine*. Orem, UT: Bi-World Publishers, 1979.

Hobbs, Christopher, D.O.M. "*Taraxacum Officinale:* A Monograph and Literature Review." *Eclectic Dispensatory*. Portland, OR: Eclectic Medical Publications, 1989.

Hoffmann, David. *The Holistic Herbal*. Findhorn, Scotland: The Findhorn Press, 1983.

Jones, Pamela. *Just Weeds*. New York: Prentice-Hall Press, 1991.

Keville, Kathi. *The Illustrated Herb Encyclopedia*. New York: Mallard Press, 1991.

Kirschmann, Gayla, and John D. Kirschmann. *Nutrition Almanac*. San Francisco: McGraw Hill, 1996.

Kotobuki Seiyaku K.K. Pat. JP 81/10117 (1981), Japan.

Krroeber, L. "Pharmacology of inulin drugs and their therapeutic use." *II Pharmazie* 5:122–127, 1950.

Lowenfield, Claire, and Philippa Back. *The Complete Book of Herbs and Spices*. Boton: Little Brown and Company, 1974.

Mabey, Richard. *The New Age Herbalist*. New York: Collier Books, 1988.

McIntyre, Anne. *Flower Power*. New York: Henry Holt and Company, 1996.

McVicar, Jekka. *Herbs for the Home*. New York: Viking Studio Books, 1994.

Meyer, Clarence. *Fifty Years of the Herbalist Almanac*. Glenwood, IL: Meyerbooks, 1977.

Mills, Simon Y. *The Essential Book of Herbal Medicine*. New York: Penguin Group, 1991.

Mills, Simon, and Steven Finando. *Alternatives in Healing*. New York: New American Library, 1988.

Mowrey, Daniel B. *Herbal Tonic Therapies*. New Canaan, CT: Keats Publishing, 1993.

Murray, Michael T., N.D. *The Healing Power of Herbs*. Rocklin, CA: Prima Publishing, 1995.

Null, Gary. *Herbs for the Seventies.* New York: Dell Books 1972.

Ody, Penelope. *The Complete Medicinal Herbal.* New York: DK Publishing, 1993.

————. *Home Herbal.* New York: DK Publishing, 1995.

Pahlow, Mannfried. *Healing Plants.* Hauppauge, NY: Barrons Publishing, 1993.

Phillips, Roger, and Nicky Foy. *The Random House Book of Herbs.* New York: Random House, 1990.

Racz-Kotilla, Elizabeth, Gabriel Racz, and A. Solomon. "The action of *Taraxacum officinale* extracts on the body weight and diuresis of laboratory animals." *Planta Medica* 26:212–7, 1974.

St. Claire, Debra. *The Herbal Medicine Cabinet.* Berkeley, CA: Celestial Arts, 1997.

Sanders, Jack. *Hedgemaids and Fairy Candles.* Camden, ME: Ragged Mountain Press, 1993.

Scully, Virginia. *A Treasury of American Indian Foods.* New York: Crown Publishers, 1972.

Stuart, Malcom. *The Encyclopedia of Herbs and Herbalism.* New York: Crescent Books, 1979.

Treben, Maria. *Health Through God's Pharmacy.* Steyer, Austria: Wilhelm Ennsthaler, 1984.

Weed, Susun. *Breast Cancer? Breast Health!* Woodstock, New York: Ash Tree Publishing, 1996.

————. *Healing Wise.* Woodstock, New York: Ash Tree Publishing, 1989.

Weiner, Michael, Ph.D. *Weiner's Herbal.* Mill Valley, CA: Quantum Books, 1990.

Weiner, Michael, Ph.D., and Janet Weiner. *Herbs that Heal.* Mill Valey, CA: Quantum Books, 1994.

Wheelwright, Edith Grey. *Medicinal Plants and Their History.* New York: Dover Publications, 1974.

Willard, Terry, Ph.D. *A Textbook of Modern Herbology.* Calgary, Canada: Progressive Publishing, 1988.

————. *The Wild Rose Scientific HerbalWild Rose.* Calgary, Canada: College of Natural Healing, 1991.

Wood, Magda Ironside. *Herbs.* Secaucus, NJ: Castle Books, 1975.

SOURCES

Defenders of Dandelion

The Defenders of Dandelion organization can be contacted at:

Goosefoot Acres
P.O. Box 18016
Cleveland, OH 44118
1-800-697-4858
To become a member of Defenders of Dandelion, which includes receiving a book, T-shirt that says "Celebrate Dandelions — If you can't beat them, eat them!" or tote bag, quarterly newsletter subscription, bumper sticker, and 10% off all products, send $35 plus $3.50 postage and handling. You can also get a free product catalog.

Dandelion Festivals

For information on Vineland's yearly Dandelion Festival, contact the Vineland Chamber of Commerce:
P.O. Box 489
Vineland, NJ 08360
(800) 309-0019

Dandelion Seeds

For dandelion seeds, try any of the following mail-order sources.

Horizon Herbs
P.O. Box 69
Williams, OR 97544-0069
(541) 846-6704

Abundant Life Seed Foundation
P.O. Box 772
Port Townsend, WA 98368
(206) 385-5660

Organic Herbs
Trout Lake Farm
149 Little Mountain Road
Trout Lake, WA 988650
(509) 395-2025

Fresh and Dried Herbs

If you can't gather your own and don't have a local source, you can always obtain dried dandelion leaves and roots from mail-order herb shops such as those listed here.

Blessed Herbs
109 Barre Plains Road
Oakham, MA 01068
(508) 882-3839

Jean's Greens
119 Sulphur Spring Road
Norway, NY 13416
(888) 845-TEAS
Fax: (315) 845-6501
Web site: www.jeansgreens.com

Mountain Rose Herbs
20818 High Street
North San Juan, CA 95960
 (800) 879-3337
Fax: (530) 292-9138
Web site:
    www.botanical.com/mtrose

Penn Herb Company, Ltd.
10601 Decatur Road, Suite 2
Philadelphia, PA 19154
(215) 632-6100

Sage Woman Herbs
2211 West Colorado Avenue
Colorado Springs, CO 80904
(719) 473-9702
Fax: (719) 473-8873

Nature's Herb Company
47444 Kato Road
Fremont, CA 94538
(510) 651-4591

Sunrise Herb Company
4808 Dreams End Drive
Louisville, KY 40291
(888) 880-0384

INDEX

Entries in **boldface** indicate recipes. Page references in **boldface** indicate charts, and those in *italics* indicate illustrations.

From: _____

BUSINESS REPLY MAIL

FIRST-CLASS MAIL   PERMIT NO. 2   POWNAL VT

POSTAGE WILL BE PAID BY ADDRESSEE

STOREY'S BOOKS FOR COUNTRY LIVING
STOREY COMMUNICATIONS INC
RR1 BOX 105
POWNAL VT 05261-9988

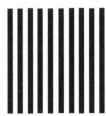

We'd love your thoughts . . .

Your reactions, criticisms, things you did or didn't like about this Storey Book. Please use space below (or write a letter if you'd prefer — even send photos!) telling how you've made use of the information . . . how you've put it to work . . . the more details the better!

Thanks in advance for your help in building our library of good Storey Books.

Pamela B. Art
Publisher, Storey Books

Book Title: _____

Purchased From: _____

Comments: _____

_____

_____

_____

_____

_____

Your Name: _____

Mailing Address: _____

E-mail Address: _____

☐ Please check here if you'd like our latest Storey's Books for Country Living Catalog.

☐ You have my permission to quote from my comments and use these quotations in ads, brochures, mail, and other promotions used to market Storey Books.

Signed _____ Date _____

e-mail=feedback@storey.com   www.storey.com   PRINTED IN THE USA   4/99

OTHER STOREY TITLES YOU WILL ENJOY

Herbal Antibiotics, by Stephen Harrod Buhner. Also in Storey's Medicinal Herb Guide series, this book presents all the current information about antibiotic-resistant microbes and the herbs that are most effective in fighting them. Readers will also find detailed, step-by-step instructions for making and using herbal infusions, tinctures, teas, and salves to treat various types of infections. 144 pages. Paperback. ISBN 1-58017-148-6.

The Herbal Home Remedy Book, by Joyce A. Wardwell. In this guide, readers will discover how to use 25 common herbs to make simple herbal remedies. Native American legends and folklore are spread throughout the book. 176 pages. Paperback. 1-58017-016-1.

Natural First Aid: Herbal Treatments for Ailments and Injuries; Emergency Preparedness; Wilderness Safety, by Brigitte Mars. Also in Storey's Medicinal Herb Guide series, this book offers quick, effective, and natural first aid suggestions for everything from ant bites to wounds. Include recipes for simple home remedies and recommends for a stocking a first aid kit for home or travel. 128 pages. Paperback. ISBN: 1-58017-147-8.

Rosemary Gladstar's Herbs for Longevity and Well-Being, by Rosemary Gladstar. A thorough exploration of the life-extending properties of herbs such as gingko, ginseng, and echinacea, and their use in cultures around the world. Includes recipes to enhance quality of life, and tips for extending life through health living. 80 pages. Paperback. ISBN 1-58017-154-0.

Saw Palmetto for Men & Women, by David Winston. Another title in Storey's Medicinal Herb Guide series. Respected herbalist Winston brings a new perspective to using this popular herb for both men's and women's health problems such as prostate enlargement, male baldness, ovarian pain and cysts, infertility, cystic acne, anorexia, and as a booster for the immune system. 128 pages. Paperback. ISBN 1-58017-206-7.

These books and other Storey Books are available at your bookstore, farm store, garden center, or directly from Storey Books, Schoolhouse Road, Pownal, Vermont 05261, or by calling 1-800-441-5700. Or visit our Web site at www.storey.com.